You Should NEVER Walk Alone

The Story of Hoz Neurosurgery Mentorship

Editors

Rania H. Al-Taie

Samer S. Hoz

You Should NEVER Walk Alone

The Story of Hoz Neurosurgery Mentorship

Editors

Rania H. Al-Taie
Mustansiriyah University, College of Medicine, Baghdad, Iraq.
Email: raniahussain03@gmail.com

Samer S. Hoz
Department of of Neurosurgery, University of Cincinnati Medical Center, Cincinnati, United States.
Email: hozsamer2055@gmail.com

Foreword

It gives me great pleasure to write a foreword for this special and unique book, *"You Should Never Walk Alone."* This book came to life through years of hard work through the Hoz Neurosurgery Mentorship Program. It has helped guide medical students and young doctors from Iraq and other countries to become future leaders in medicine, research, and innovation.

Mentorship in medicine dates to the Islamic Golden Age, when renowned doctors such as Al-Razi (Rhazes) and Ibn Sina (Avicenna) taught their students not only medical knowledge but also good values and ethics. In modern times, mentorship has become more organized, thanks to Sir William Osler, often regarded as the father of modern medical education.

Dr. Samer Hoz initiated his Mentorship Program in Iraq, despite limited resources and high hopes. The program shows that the best investment is in people. As the book wisely says, *"The mentor is not the one who creates doctors; he is the one who provides them with the opportunity to create themselves."* This means a real mentor helps others discover their strengths and become their best.

This book is special because it is written by young doctors who have personally experienced these challenges. They share true stories about the hard times they faced, what they learned, and how they reached their goals. Their stories show how support, teamwork, and dedication can build a better future for medicine.

As you read this book, I hope you feel the hard work in every story. I would like to express my appreciation to the dedicated editors Rania H. Al-Taie and Samer S. Hoz, and to all the contributors whose efforts and inspiring experiences have enriched this remarkable work and made it a valuable guide for future generations.

A Hadi Al Khalili, MD
Former head of the Department of Neurosurgery,
Neurosurgeon at College of Medicine - University of Baghdad
Baghdad University, Iraq

Foreword

The book you will start reading is one of the few in medical literature devoted to mentoring. Every mentor is a tutor, but not every tutor is a mentor. While tutors guide your steps with precious technical pearls that help you flawlessly complete a surgery, a mentor is a tutor who goes one step beyond the specifics of that day. A mentor recognizes in your performance as a trainee characteristic that the mentor perceived need to be refined or supported to allow you to grow from a technical surgeon into an innovative surgeon. It is possible to recognize the tutors of a generation of surgeons, but mentees of the same mentor are different. Tutors train you vertically; mentors train you horizontally.

The chapter "Foundations of the Mentorship Program" mentions that mentor is an eponym of Mentor, a character from Homer's poems where we are told that Odysseus, before departing for war and sensing that he may be many years away from home, confided the care of his son Telemachus to his good friend Mentor. Odysseus's trusted Mentor to guide Telemachus through his formative years. All along the twenty years of Odysseus' absence from Ithaca, it was from Mentor's lessons that Telemachus gained the confidence to face the suitors who pretended to marry his mother under the assumption that Odysseus would not return. Through the confidence in himself that Mentor installed in him, Telemachus sailed away from Ithaca in search of his father. The figure of Mentor was so strong that the goddess Athenea transformed herself into Mentor when advising Telemachus.

You may ask why I brought a fictitious character into the book's foreword addressed to clinical scientists. But this is a book, where the authors share their experiences with an outstanding mentor.

I advise you to read it paying attention to the feelings between the lines. You will notice a relationship between the Mentor and the mentees that is like two-way lane between the senior and the juniors, a two-way road with heavy traffic of confidence and trust between the characters of this beautiful epic poem that is medical education.

Jorge A. Lazaref
Professor Emeritus of pediatric neurosurgeon,
UCLA Medical Center, Santa Monica
Ronald Reagan UCLA Medical Center
Los Angeles, California., USA.

Foreword

"Samer, everything has stopped.
The pandemic has paralyzed everything.
UpSurgeOn is done.
Would you be open to me sending you some cranial simulators?
At least we'll be doing something useful in your lab, for your students."

He didn't hesitate.
"Absolutely. Do it."

I'll never forget that phone call. It was April 2021, and everything felt like it was falling apart.

Just three months earlier, we had launched the very first simulation technologies developed by a young medtech startup called UpSurgeOn—a project I had founded with a small team of doctors, designers, and engineers few years before. Our goal was ambitious: to reimagine neurosurgical training through physical simulators and virtual technologies. An idea born from deep frustration, after years of witnessing how inaccessible surgical education was for so many around the world.

At that time, UpSurgeOn was still a fragile experiment. A few passionate people. A tiny lab in Milan. Two years of intense development behind us… and then, just as we launched the very first simulators, the world stopped.

Hospitals shifted into emergency mode. Surgical training was no longer a priority. Operating rooms were shut down, and neurosurgeons — myself included — were reassigned to COVID wards.

In the mornings, I worked hospital shifts in full protective gear. In the evenings, I sat alone in the UpSurgeOn workspace, asking myself if everything we had built was about to disappear. The technologies were ready — but no one was interested in using them in that moment. Our team was anxious, lost, paralyzed. The dream we had fought for suddenly felt irrelevant.

That's when I called Samer.

We had met years earlier through an international WhatsApp group — Neurosurgery Grand Rounds — one of those rare digital spaces where borders dissolve, and people connect through shared passion. It was around 2016. Samer was already an experienced neurosurgeon. I was finishing my residency. But he never made me feel the difference. He listened, he shared, he cared. And in that connection, I recognized something rare: vision grounded in action.

That's why, years later, in that surreal April of 2021, I picked up the phone and told him what we were going through. I needed to connect with the most visionary and open-minded colleague I knew. And Samer Hoz was the very first person who came to mind.

Within days, we shipped two boxes of cranial simulators to the Hoz Lab, Samer's neurosurgical training center in Baghdad. And just a few days later, he organized a wonderful course.

That moment changed everything.

It became the first cadaver-free neurosurgery course in the world, held in one of the most challenging regions on Earth, right in the middle of a global pandemic. Social media lit up. People from every corner of the planet were talking about it.

That improvised, desperate gesture — packing up simulation technologies and shipping them across the globe — became our operating model. And I realized something I'll never forget: Technology alone means nothing. You need people bold enough to build magic around it.

The truth is — I didn't know how to use those simulators. I didn't know how to create that magic.

The Hoz Lab showed us the way. It was there that the very first spark happened. They created the first magic.

In the six months that followed, we ran 12 courses in 12 countries where access to surgical training was limited or nonexistent. Over the next three years, we delivered 45 free neurosurgery courses, writing a new chapter in the history of surgical education.

There were brain aneurysms clipped by trainees on four different continents — the same aneurysm, the same course, reproduced in vastly different settings. One day, the same simulation was happening simultaneously at the Mayo Clinic and in Ethiopia.
A global community was beginning to form.

UpSurgeOn grew rapidly — from a fragile idea to a global medtech company, now operating in more than 110 countries, across four surgical specialties.

And all of it — started with the Hoz Lab, and the spark of magic they revealed to the world.

The Hoz Lab is not just a facility. It's a declaration. Born in a country marked by challenges, it represents a powerful idea: education doesn't wait for ideal conditions — it grows through courage, resilience, and belief.

At the Hoz Lab, surgical education isn't about fancy equipment — it's about training a new mindset. It's about giving young surgeons the opportunity to learn and guide innovation at the same time.

The most moving moment for me came when Samer invited me to speak to his students.
From that point forward, our collaboration grew. We wrote together, shared experiences, and built new visions. I discovered a generation that would do anything to help their country.
They didn't to compromise — they wanted to transform it. They believed in the dignity of knowledge. I felt their maturity, their openness, and their deep awareness that life is not always perfect — but that it is worth living if you dedicate yourself to making it better.

This book is not just the story of a lab that trains surgical trainees.
It is the story of a man who chose to resist by creating cultural magic. A man who built a lab not just to train hands — but to awaken minds. To inspire a new generation of thinkers, innovators, and free spirits. It is a story about bold decisions, impossible odds, and the transformative power of belief.

Today, the Hoz Lab stands as a beacon for all those who believe that knowledge is a right, not a privilege. And if there's one thing I've learned from all of this, it's that: When education becomes an act of courage, no border can stop it.

This foreword is my personal testimony to a beautiful creation, and my deep gratitude for having had the chance to witness it.

Federico Nicolosi
Consultant Neurosurgeon, Department of neurosurgery,
Humanitas Research Hospital, Milan. Italy
Founder and CEO of UpSurgeOn
Member of WFNS – Young Neurosurgeons Committee

Preface

To me, this book is a deeply personal milestone. As someone who has lived through every phase of this mentorship journey. From the early days of dreaming and drafting to the intense, often emotional process of building a community. I felt a responsibility to put this story into words. It is a story that deserves to be remembered, one that captures what we achieved and why it mattered.

The decision to document this mentorship journey came from a strong belief that stories like these matter. I wanted to reflect on the progress we made, the obstacles we faced, and the small, often unnoticed victories that shaped our collective growth. Every chapter is a reminder of what can happen when people come together around a shared purpose.

I am proud of what we accomplished. It started with an idea and evolved into a community. An environment where students could be challenged, supported, and seen. Along the way, I witnessed transformation, both in others and in myself. This program helped shape who I am, and writing about it helped me understand just how far we've come.

I hope this book finds its way into the hands of those who are searching for guidance, reassurance, or an example of what can be achieved when passion meets purpose. If this story ignites a spark in even one reader, encouraging them to mentor, to lead, or to dream—then it has fulfilled its purpose.

Because the greatest journeys are never meant to be walked alone.

Rania H. Al-Taie

Key features

- In-depth exploration of neurosurgery mentorship programs, highlighting the critical role mentorship plays in shaping the skills, professional development, and personal growth of mentees in the medical field.
- Comprehensive analysis of the development and evolution of neurosurgery in resource-limited settings, with a focus on overcoming challenges such as technological limitations and access to advanced surgical training.
- Detailed insights into practical aspect of the mentorship, including surgical simulations, case studies, and hands-on neurosurgical training designed to enhance technical precision and clinical decision-making.
- Real examples demonstrating the impact of mentorship programs on career trajectories, skill enhancement, and research productivity, providing a blueprint for developing future mentorship initiatives.
- Global perspectives on mentorship in neurosurgery, focusing on international collaboration, and the integration of advanced technologies.
- Practical guidelines for implementing mentorship programs in diverse medical settings, with a focus on sustainability, scalability, and adapting to varying levels of resource availability.
- Discussion on the importance of fostering teamwork, leadership, and continuous learning in neurosurgery mentorship, ensuring the growth of future medical professionals.

Content list:

List of contributors	
Author	**Affiliation**
Aktham O. Al-Khafaji	University of Baghdad, College of Medicine, Baghdad, Iraq
Ahmed Muthana	university of Baghdad, college of medicine, Baghdad, Iraq
Ali A. Dolachee	Department of Surgery, Al-Kindy College of Medicine, University of Baghdad, Baghdad, Iraq
Ali M. Neamah	College of Medicine, University of Baghdad, IRAQ
Alkawthar M. Abdulsada	neurosurgery teaching hospital, Baghdad, Iraq
Bandar M. Alhadeethi	University of Baghdad, College of Medicine, Baghdad, Iraq
Fatimah Oday Ahmed	Al-Mustansiriyah University College of Medicine, Baghdad, Iraq
Hagar A. Algburi	Medical student, College of Medicine, University of Baghdad. Baghdad, Iraq.
Haneen A. Salih	– Department of Molecular and Medical Biotechnology, College of Biotechnology, Al-Nahrain University, Baghdad, Iraq. – Department of Biology, University of Al-Mustansiriyah, College of Sciences, Baghdad, Iraq.
JaaferAbdulWahid	Al-Nahrain University, College Of Medicine, Baghdad, Iraq
Mahmood F. Al-Zaidy	College of Medicine, University of Baghdad, IRAQ
Mohammed A Al-Dhahir	University of Florida-College of Medicine-Department of Neuroscience, USA
Mohammed S. Al-Baldawi	College of Medicine, University of Anbar, Anbar, Iraq.
Mustafa Ayad Murayati	College of Medicine, University of Baghdad, Baghdad, Iraq
Nedal Abusedra	Neurosurgery Department, Albasheer Hospital, Amman, Jordan
Noor Al-Saadi	University of Babylon-College of Medicine, Hilla, Iraq
Rania H. Al-Taie	College of Medicine, University of Mustansiriyah, Baghdad, Iraq.
Rokaya H. Abdalridha	Babylon University/College of Medicine Babylon, Iraq
Saja Amer Albanaa	Department of Surgery, University of Baghdad, College of Medicine

Sama S. Albairmani	Neurosurgery Department, Al-Iraqia University, College of Medicine, Baghdad, Iraq
Samer S. Hoz	Department of Neurosurgery, University of Cincinnati Medical Center, Cincinnati, OH, USA
Sura H Talib	Department of surgery, College of Medicine, University of Al-Mustansiriyah, Baghdad, IRAQ
Teeba A. Al-Ageely	Department of Neurosurgery, University of Baghdad, Baghdad, Iraq.
Younus M. Al-Khazaali	College of Medicine, Al-Nahrain University, Baghdad, Iraq.
Zinah A. Al-Araji	Alnahrain university, college of medicine

Dedication

"To Rabab F. Mohammed, Hussein A. Al-Taie, Malak H. Al-Taie, and Yaceen H. Al-Taie. Because of your love, strength, and belief in me, I never walked alone. And to my mentor, whose guidance shaped my journey and whose unwavering faith made me who I am today.
This book carries your spirit on every page." **Rania H. Al-Taie**

"To my lovely family: Sawsan, Saad, Arwa, Farah, Ward, Samhar, Anoona, Sanaa, Faris, and Luay. To the best mentors Prof. Alkhalili, Prof. Ausman, Prof. Lazarref, Dr. Matti, Prof. Andaluz, and Prof. Prestigiacomo". **Samer S. Hoz**

Introduction to the Book: You Should NEVER Walk Alone

In every great story of achievement, there lies a pivotal moment when the right guidance and support unlock unimaginable potential. This book tells that story not just about neurosurgery but also about personal growth, resilience, and the transformative power of mentorship. It seeks to document the journey of the Hoz Neurosurgery Mentorship Program, an initiative born from a desire to uplift, empower, and guide young medical professionals toward their dreams.

This book is not about telling our story but is a comprehensible mentorship model that shaped careers, enriched lives, and enthused future leaders. The success of careers as complex and demanding as neurosurgery is seldom enjoyed alone. The weight of medical practice, the intricacies of surgery, and the emotional challenges in patient care are best negotiated with the wisdom and encouragement of mentors who have walked the path before them.

The program was initiated to bridge the gap between aspiration and accomplishment and helped scores of students and professionals enhance their skills, knowledge, and confidence to grow fully. This mentorship provides one-to-one guidance, hands-on practice, and a positive atmosphere for cooperation and independent thinking.

Each chapter discusses the mentorship model and key elements throughout this book, offering insights into the structure of how mentee professional pathways have taken shape. Also, we introduce global perspectives interwoven throughout the program that provide a unique insight into how mentorship can be applied to a variety of cultural and often resource-limited settings.

The Hoz Neurosurgery Mentorship Program is a product of dedication, passion, and a belief that medical education should transcend textbooks and exams. It should inspire, challenge, and transform. This book serves as a guide on how to establish mentorship initiatives that are both sustainable and impactful, especially in environments where resources may be scarce but the desire to learn is abundant.

Whether you are a student or a mentor desiring to create change in medical education, we invite you on this journey. It is a model that has made us witness how mentees grow into confident professionals and then, in turn, become mentors themselves to further propagate the chain of support, knowledge-sharing, and compassion.

This book is more than a record of accomplishments; it is an invitation to rethink how we train, support, and empower the next generation of medical professionals. Together, we can create mentorship experiences that truly elevate the careers and lives of those who dare to dream.

Section 1: Foundations of the Mentorship Program

CH.1: Defining the Vision and Core Objectives of the Hoz Mentorship Program

Rania H. Al-Taie, Hagar A. Algburi, Mohammed S. Al-Baldawi, Teeba A. Al-Ageely

Section 1: Foundations of the Mentorship Program

CH.1: Defining the Vision and Core Objectives of the Hoz Mentorship Program

Mentorship has long stood as a cornerstone of surgical education, transcending generations and geographical boundaries. William Halstead, regarded as the architect of the modern surgical residency, embedded the Socratic method into a structured, immersive model of training, emphasizing graduated responsibility and deep clinical immersion [1]. His impact extended beyond curriculum design; it was philosophical, shaping generations of surgeons through a rigorous yet intimate educational process. Among those influenced by this method was Harvey Cushing, the founder of neurosurgery as a specialty. Cushing's development was profoundly shaped by two mentors, William Osler and Halstead himself, both of whom invested in him not only surgical wisdom but also the temperament and intellectual depth required to pioneer a new field [2].

However, mentorship is not the invention of modern academia. The very term "mentor" finds its roots in ancient Greek mythology. In Homer's Odyssey, when Odysseus left for the Trojan War, he entrusted the care of his son, Telemachus, to "Mentor", a wise and faithful companion who was later revealed to be the goddess Athena in disguise. The mentor's role was not to instruct Telemachus in a narrow skill but to guide his maturation, instill virtue, and foster independence. This archetype of mentorship as a holistic, character-centered relationship has endured across centuries and cultures [3].

In ancient Greece, it was customary for youth to be assigned mentors who would guide them through not only the acquisition of knowledge but also the absorption of cultural values, ethical reasoning, and philosophical inquiry [3]. This immersive model of learning through imitation, reflection, and trust laid the groundwork for the evolution of teaching in arts, sciences, and medicine. Zuckerman's seminal work on the genealogy of Nobel laureates underscores this point. Among 92 laureates studied, 48 had trained under previous laureates [4]. What bound these relationships was not merely the transfer of expertise, but the imparting of a distinctive intellectual ethos, a "style of thinking" that transcended formal instruction.

In contemporary surgical training, this historical blueprint continues to unfold. A successful mentor-mentee relationship is profoundly synergistic. It is not a one-way transmission of knowledge but a dynamic interplay of trust, vulnerability, and mutual aspiration. Mentees learn to navigate not only clinical complexity but also the nuanced terrain of professional life. They benefit from honest, unfiltered feedback and are offered a rare glimpse into the informal rules of career advancement, research productivity, and institutional navigation [3]. The mentor, in turn, experiences a powerful form of professional renewal. Through the mentee's growth, the mentor re-engages with their own sense of purpose, sharpens their own thinking, and contributes to the perpetuation of excellence in the field. The process fosters a quiet but profound legacy.

The success of mentorship, however, is not automatic. It requires baseline chemistry, shared values, and mutual commitment. Trust is the currency. Respect is the foundation. And character, not merely competence, must be the focal point [3]. A mentor must have the capacity to see what a mentee does not yet see in themselves and the wisdom to know when to step forward with instruction and when to step back with belief. As Steven Spielberg so eloquently stated, "The delicate balance of mentoring someone is not creating them in your own image but giving them the opportunity to create themselves."

Yet despite the clear, time-tested value of mentorship, structured and accessible programs remain scarce, especially in low- and middle-income countries. This scarcity is not due to lack of need but due to a lack of infrastructure, time, and sometimes, belief in the feasibility of such systems. The consequence is a generation of capable, driven medical students who often find themselves adrift in a sea of complexity, left to navigate their professional journeys without the compass of experience that only a mentor can provide. Addressing this gap requires more than rhetorical support; it requires deliberate strategies to institutionalize mentorship as a central pillar of medical education.

In tracing the lineage of mentorship through the ages, one cannot overlook the Hippocratic Oath, which explicitly honors the teacher-learner relationship. Hippocrates declared: "To hold the one who has taught me this art as equal to my parents and to live my life in partnership with him" [5]. This sentiment goes beyond obligation, it reflects a moral and spiritual alliance between mentor and mentee. In modern terms, the mentor is a steward of potential, guiding the mentee toward self-actualization, professional excellence, and ethical responsibility [6].

In surgical specialties, particularly neurosurgery, the role of mentorship becomes even more vital. The technical demands, emotional stakes, and intensity of the learning curve require more than passive observation or textbook learning. Early mentorship has been shown to increase the likelihood that medical students pursue surgical careers and, more importantly, that they enter those careers with resilience, confidence, and ethical clarity [7]. For some students, mentorship becomes the defining experience of their medical training, the force that transforms uncertainty into purpose.

This chapter introduces the philosophical and structural foundations of the Hoz Neurosurgery Mentorship Program, a program born from the recognition that no student, no future surgeon, should ever walk alone. It is a model designed not only to teach surgical skills but to inspire a more profound sense of belonging, ethical identity, and professional vision. Informed by history, shaped by necessity, and powered by belief, the Hoz Mentorship Program aspires to uphold the noblest traditions of mentorship while addressing the urgent gaps of our present moment.

Who is a Mentor?

Defining who qualifies as a mentor in medical education, particularly in neurosurgery, is far from a straightforward task. Mentorship is not a formal title, nor is it automatically conferred by seniority or experience. It is a role that must be actively earned and continually sustained through behavior, commitment, and relational intelligence. The literature presents a wide array of definitions and expectations, reflecting a notable degree of heterogeneity across educational systems, institutional cultures, and specialties. Yet, despite this diversity, a clear consensus emerges: a true mentor embodies a triad of essential domains, personal characteristics, professional attributes, and behaviors that intentionally support and uplift the mentee.

A mentor is not merely a more experienced practitioner who teaches procedural steps or shares clinical cases. Rather, a mentor is a transformational figure. Someone who empowers the mentee to explore their identity, overcome their limitations, and pursue mastery with courage and clarity. In the surgical context, this role becomes even more critical. Surgery is not just a skill set; it is a discipline that requires resilience, humility, decisiveness, and unwavering ethical integrity. These cannot be acquired from textbooks or observed passively in operating theaters. They must be transmitted, modeled, and reinforced through meaningful human connection.

A mentor walks alongside, neither leading from above nor pushing from behind but standing shoulder-to-shoulder with the learner through moments of uncertainty, failure, and discovery. This relational dynamic is not accidental. It is built on trust, mutual respect, and shared purpose.

Sir Isaac Newton's profound reflection— "If I have seen further, it is only by standing on the shoulders of giants" [8]—is emblematic of the mentor-mentee paradigm. In surgery, progress is built layer by layer upon the work of those who came before. The mentee ascends, not in isolation, but through the vision and elevation offered by their mentor. But with elevation comes responsibility. A mentor does not merely boost a student's perspective. They shape how that student will think, lead, and innovate.

The qualities that define an effective mentor are multidimensional. Beyond mastery of surgical techniques or academic accolades, a mentor must exhibit emotional intelligence, humility, and the patience to nurture growth at variable paces. They provide room for failure as a critical step toward success and encourage autonomy while remaining a reliable source of guidance. Table 1 outlines key characteristics such as self-awareness, credibility, accessibility, communication, and empathy, each essential in cultivating a meaningful mentor-mentee bond.

Mentors must also be inclusive and open-minded, recognizing that each mentee arrives with a unique constellation of skills, motivations, and challenges. An excellent mentor understands when to challenge and when to support when to step forward with instruction, and when to stand back and let the mentee lead. This adaptability fosters a safe learning environment in which mentees can test their limits, build resilience, and grow in confidence.

In the ever-evolving landscape of medical education, mentorship plays a foundational role not just in technical formation but in the holistic shaping of future leaders. It is not merely a teaching method. It is a philosophy of human development. The mentor must invest their time and energy without the expectation of immediate return, knowing that the seeds they plant today will bear fruit in the health systems, research breakthroughs, and patient outcomes of tomorrow. As the saying goes, "A leader is one who creates more leaders, not followers." In the world of surgery, where each decision carries immense consequences, and each procedure can alter the course of a life, the presence of a great mentor can shape not just a career but a legacy.

Table 1: Core Traits of an Effective Mentor in Medical Education [3, 9].

Trait	Description	How it Impacts Mentees
Self-awareness	Recognizing one's own strengths, weaknesses, and biases to mentor with integrity and insight.	Builds trust and models reflective practice for mentees.
Professional credibility	Possessing expertise, qualifications, and recognition in the field; serving as a role model.	Inspires confidence and sets a benchmark for professional excellence.
Organizational insight	Understanding institutional dynamics, resources, and strategies for career navigation.	Helps mentees access hidden opportunities and avoid systemic pitfalls.
Time commitment	Regularly dedicating time for guidance, feedback, and support despite professional demands.	Reinforces mentees' sense of value and fosters reliability in the relationship.
Communication skills	Active listening, clear articulation, and the ability to adapt language to the mentee's level.	Enhances understanding, reduces miscommunication, and strengthens connection.
Empowerment	Creating safe spaces for mentees to try, fail, reflect, and grow without fear of judgment.	Boosts confidence, resilience, and independence.
Developmental orientation	A deep commitment to helping others grow intellectually, professionally, and personally.	Enables mentees to clarify goals and align efforts with long-term development.
Innovative thinking	Being open to new perspectives, methods, and solutions in mentorship and clinical training.	Encourages creativity and adaptability among mentees.
Empathy	Understanding and validating the mentee's challenges, emotions, and perspectives.	Builds psychological safety and emotional resilience.
Cultural sensitivity	Acknowledging and respecting the diverse backgrounds, identities, and values of mentees.	Promotes inclusivity and helps mentees feel seen and respected in all their dimensions.

The Measurable Role of Mentorship in Surgical Education and Advancement

The advancement of mentorship programs within academic medical institutions must begin with a deep understanding of their measurable impact. Numerous studies have demonstrated that mentorship significantly influences the academic success, career trajectory, research engagement, and clinical competence of medical students. However, there remains a considerable gap between the acknowledged value of mentorship and its actual availability.

A compelling survey revealed that while 95% of medical students regard mentorship as essential to their academic and professional development, only 33% report having meaningful access to a mentor [10]. This disparity highlights a systemic underutilization of mentorship as a strategic educational intervention, especially concerning the increasing complexity of medical training and the rising competitiveness of residency placements.

In surgical specialties, particularly those as demanding as neurosurgery, orthopedics, and plastic surgery, the role of mentorship is even more pronounced. As residency positions become more limited, mentorship emerges as a decisive factor influencing both application strength and specialty selection. Notably, the majority of surgical residents report forming mentorship relationships during the pre-clinical years of their training, a period often overlooked in structured mentorship planning [11]. Furthermore, nearly 80% of students pursuing careers in plastic or orthopedic surgery attribute their specialty choice to the influence of a mentor, underscoring the mentor's role not only as an educator but as a career shaper and source of inspiration [10].

Another critical dimension of mentorship is its potential to correct disparities in access and representation within the medical workforce. Diversity in mentorship program design is not simply a matter of inclusion, it is a strategic imperative. Students from underrepresented racial, ethnic, and socioeconomic backgrounds often face greater barriers to entry and advancement within surgical specialties [14]. Targeted mentorship can bridge these gaps by providing tailored guidance, equitable access to opportunities, and culturally competent support systems. Studies indicate that mentorship enhances the pipeline of diverse candidates into surgery and has downstream benefits for patient care, particularly in underserved communities [10].

However, current trends reveal persistent inequities. Women, for instance, are statistically less likely to receive mentorship in surgical fields and remain underrepresented in academic medicine, especially in leadership positions [12].

In recent years, the emphasis on research experience, letters of recommendation, and sponsorship has escalated within residency application processes. These elements have become key differentiators for candidates, especially in competitive specialties. According to the Association of American Medical Colleges (AAMC), the number of students taking a dedicated research year during medical school more than doubled between 1995 and 2010 [13]. For instance, nearly one-third of applicants to orthopedic surgery programs now complete a research year, using this time to strengthen their portfolios and forge deeper connections with faculty mentors.

Research involvement offers multifaceted benefits. It enhances the student's scientific literacy, provides mentors with insight into the mentee's dedication and capability, and allows for the cultivation of long-term academic collaborations. Mentors who work with students across various clinical and research environments, such as operating rooms, clinics, and academic settings, are uniquely positioned to write detailed, personalized, and impactful letters of recommendation. These letters often carry significant weight in residency selection committees, as they speak to the applicant's clinical reasoning, professionalism, teamwork, and resilience.

Furthermore, mentorship can evolve into sponsorship, a deeper level of advocacy in which mentors actively utilize their networks and reputation to promote the mentee's opportunities. This may include directly contacting program directors to recommend a student for a research position, advocating during residency interviews, or recommending mentees for fellowships and professional societies [10]. While mentorship supports development, sponsorship opens doors.

In summary, the data is precise. Structured mentorship programs are not ancillary to medical education; they are essential. With thoughtful integration, mentorship can elevate training outcomes, reduce inequities, and transform potential into excellence.

Why I Shouldn't Be Alone?

Nature offers compelling metaphors for the power of connection. The unity of a wolf pack, the tireless cooperation of worker bees, and the shared intelligence of ant colonies all reflect a truth that transcends species, survival and progress are collective endeavors. While human beings may consider themselves more advanced, gifted with intellect, adaptability, and complex emotional lives, we are no less reliant on one another. Consider the proverb where a single stick may break with ease, but a bundle is near impossible to bend. In medicine, this principle is not symbolic. It is operational.

Ambition and competitiveness often drive medical students to excel. These traits are, without question, powerful motivators. Yet, in the absence of collaboration, they can evolve into isolation, burnout, and diminished capacity. The pressure to stand out can paradoxically separate students from the very community that sustains them. In surgical settings, individual decisions can indeed be lifesaving. But no decision is enacted in a vacuum. Even the most heroic act in the operating room is scaffolded by teamwork, coordination, and collective vigilance.

Reaching the top of your field is an admirable goal, but the summit is lonelier without those who climbed beside you. There is a deeper satisfaction in rising together, lifting others as you ascend. This is not only the ethos of medicine but its practical necessity. A shared journey builds trust, resilience, and lasting purpose. Collaboration transforms milestones into memories and ambition into shared legacy.

Collaborative learning environments cultivate not only productivity but also a shared sense of mission. When students with diverse perspectives and skill sets unite, they are more likely to develop creative, integrative solutions. Questions are answered more efficiently, problems are approached with multidimensional insights, and confidence is distributed rather than hoarded. Medical education, particularly in resource-constrained or highly competitive environments, poses daunting challenges, including time limitations, high costs of clinical rotations, and restricted access to hands-on training. Facing these hurdles in isolation increases the likelihood of discouragement or failure. However, facing them in a community setting invites adaptation, encouragement, and shared strategy.

Mentorship plays a pivotal role in this dynamic. Studies have consistently shown that mentored students adapt more easily to the demands of medical education, benefit from strategic career planning, and demonstrate higher research productivity [14–16]. A skilled mentor helps students distinguish between visionary and practical goals, recognizing strengths and weaknesses that may elude the mentee's self-perception. Based on experience and insight, the mentor can help design a structured plan that is individualized, measurable, achievable, relevant, and time-bound. A personalized blueprint for growth.

The psychological underpinnings of these needs are well-established. According to Maslow's hierarchy of needs, the desire for connection, belonging, and affiliation is not a luxury. It is foundational [17]. Once basic needs for safety and stability are met, the human psyche seeks companionship, acceptance, and identity within a group. In high-stakes fields like surgery, where pressure and emotional fatigue are constant companions, the absence of social support can undermine both cognitive performance and emotional well-being. Maslow warned that individuals deprived of meaningful relationships may become psychologically fragmented, regardless of their competence or intelligence. In surgical training, being alone is not a neutral state. It is a liability.

Emerging neuroscientific data reinforces this truth at a biological level. Loneliness is not just a psychological or emotional state; it is a measurable neurophysiological condition that alters brain function and architecture. Chronic loneliness is associated with structural and functional changes in the medial prefrontal cortex, anterior insula, amygdala, and hippocampus—regions essential for emotional regulation, social cognition, and executive functioning [18]. These neural changes mimic those seen in clinical depression, anxiety disorders, and even the early stages of Alzheimer's disease. Functional MRI studies show that loneliness disturbs activity in the default mode network and attentional systems, impairing a person's ability to read social cues, regulate emotion, and make decisions under stress [18]. In other words, loneliness doesn't just feel bad; it affects how we think, relate, and respond.

In the surgical world, where split-second decisions, emotional resilience, and team dynamics can mean the difference between life and death, being neurologically compromised by social disconnection can have profound implications. Humans are, at their core, biologically wired for connection. In medicine, and especially in surgery, the mentor-mentee relationship and peer support are not optional.

To walk this path alone is to ignore the very structure of your brain, the nature of your profession, and the heart of your humanity.

Pearls from Mentees

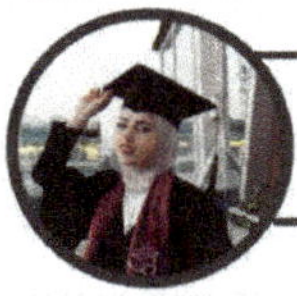

Teeba A. Al-Ageely

I believe that some coincidences shape the people we become and that the best things in life are unplanned.
During my early years in medical school, I was overwhelmed like most of my peers. Generally, goals are harder to achieve when you don't have a clear vision of what you want to do in the future, everyone said that it was too soon to tell, and although that was partly true, there's nothing wrong with addressing a few things early. I achieved a good level of basic college education. I was interested in learning anatomy like most young medical students, and I was interested in neuroscience during my second year, yet I felt like it was a far dream, and I feared that it was too difficult for my level at the time. I also had a passion for writing, but I always assumed that I had to let it go since I couldn't integrate it into my field.
During my third year, I was coincidentally introduced to the Hoz neurosurgery mentorship program, and after much thought, fear, and excitement, I enrolled and contacted Dr. Hoz. I still remember the first meeting I attended; I was mesmerized by this inspiring person and the hope he gave with every story. I didn't even sense the time passing by. After that, I tried my best to take every opportunity presented to me without letting stress hold me back as it did before. I learned so much about neurosurgery up close by attending surgeries, shadowing neurosurgeons, and observing patient-surgeon interactions. The months passed, and I kept trying to make use of each opportunity, even if I didn't know much about it, because at some point, I realized that that was the main objective: experiencing things I wasn't familiar with and didn't have it in my plan, and finding my passion along the way.
Randomly, a few months later, during a presentation I helped work on, Dr. Hoz asked me to be a part of a research project with the team and do the thing I like most: write about this topic. That paper was later published, and the rest is history.
I graduated from medical school with over 25 publications and with confidence and clear goals for what's next. That was an achievement I'll always be proud of, I'll always be grateful for my mentor who introduced me to my dream, supported me, and guided me through the way to achieve it.
Meeting Dr. Hoz was the beginning of something that improved so much in my academic life. I consider myself very lucky to have a mentor who can steer my passion in the right direction. This experience has been a personal growth journey as much as academic development, being in this mentorship made me gain so much confidence and teamwork principles. And I realized there's no limit to how much you can achieve when you're not doing it alone.

The History and The Current Status of Neurosurgery in Iraq

The roots of neurosurgery in Iraq stretch far beyond the modern surgical era, embedded in one of the most intellectually advanced civilizations of the ancient world. The Babylonians, who flourished in Mesopotamia nearly 4,000 years ago, demonstrated remarkable observational acuity in their documentation of neurological disorders [19]. Though couched in spiritual and supernatural interpretations, their clinical insights remain strikingly accurate by today's standards.

A Babylonian clay tablet which is currently preserved at the British Museum, offers detailed accounts of epilepsy and stroke, including descriptions of auras, seizure triggers, interictal behavior, and postictal phenomena. In one remarkable passage, a unilateral focal motor seizure is described with precision: "If at the time of his possession, while he is sitting down, his (left) eye moves to the side, a lip puckers, saliva flows from his mouth, and his hand, leg and trunk on the left side jerk (or twitch) like a newly slaughtered sheep—it is 'miqtu' (epilepsy)..." This passage reflects an early attempt to systematically observe neurological conditions, even when explained through the lens of demonic possession [19].

The formalization of neurosurgery as a medical specialty in Iraq began much later, in the mid-20th century. In the 1950s, Dr. Najeeb Al-Yaaqubi, a general surgeon, performed what is believed to be the first elective neurosurgical operation in the country. However, it was not until 1966 that neurosurgery began to take shape as a defined clinical and academic discipline. Among the most influential figures in this transformative era was Dr. Saad Al-Witry, widely regarded as the "father of modern neurosurgery in Iraq" [19]. A visionary in both practice and leadership, Dr. Al-Witry mastered a wide array of neurosurgical procedures and set unprecedented standards of excellence. Like many early pioneers in the field, Dr. Al-Witry embodied multidisciplinary expertise, serving simultaneously as neurosurgeon, neuroanesthetist, neurointensivist, and neuroradiologist for his patients [20].

In 1972, under his leadership and influence, Iraq launched its first formal neurosurgical training program. This marked a pivotal turning point with the establishment of the Neurosurgery Teaching Hospital in Baghdad, a dedicated tertiary center built with 150 beds and seven fully equipped operating theaters [20]. The early team included two senior neurosurgeons, one senior assistant, four residents, two anesthetists, and a consulting neurologist, with additional collaborative input from surrounding hospitals. The institution advanced rapidly. Within a year, Iraq's first cerebral angiography was performed, and cutting-edge technologies, including a gamma isotope scanner and a comprehensive neurophysiology unit with EMG, EEG, and 24-hour epilepsy monitoring, were introduced.

Today, the Neurosurgery Teaching Hospital continues to serve as the epicenter of neurosurgical training and service delivery in the country. It currently hosts 16 neurosurgeons, including four consultant-level specialists, and a cohort of 20 neurosurgery residents. With an annual surgical volume exceeding 2,400 operations, it remains a critical hub for the treatment of complex neurological disorders.

Nationally, Iraq now offers two accredited neurosurgical residency pathways. The Iraqi Board of Neurological Surgery, a five-year training program, is regulated by the Iraqi Medical Council. In parallel, the Arabic Board of Neurological Surgery, which spans six years, is overseen by the Arabic Medical Council. These programs reflect a commitment to harmonizing local expertise with broader regional standards of surgical training.

As of 2020, Iraq was home to 208 practicing neurosurgeons, including 7 women and 100 neurosurgery residents, among whom 17 were women —a growing but still underrepresented demographic in surgical subspecialties [19]. With a national population approaching 30 million, these numbers reflect both the progress and the continuing need for investment in neurosurgical infrastructure, gender equity, and academic expansion.

Hoz Neurosurgery Mentorship Program

In this book, we present an in-depth exploration of the Hoz Neurosurgery Mentorship Program, a transformative educational model initiated approximately seven years ago by Dr. Samer S. Hoz, a distinguished vascular neurosurgeon from Iraq. Designed to bridge the gap between academic instruction and clinical practice, this mentorship model emphasizes the holistic development of medical students and surgical residents. It aims not only to transfer technical knowledge but also to instill professional identity, critical thinking, and collaborative values essential for modern neurosurgical practice.

Throughout this work, we assess the effectiveness of the mentorship structure, examine its impact on the personal and professional growth of mentees, and analyze the practical outcomes achieved through its implementation. We also identify the key obstacles encountered during its evolution and present strategic, context-specific solutions that have allowed the program to thrive despite the challenges commonly faced in resource-constrained or conflict-affected medical systems.

The Hoz Mentorship Program was established with a clear mission: to empower medical students and early-career surgical trainees in identifying and reaching their professional goals. It rests on the belief that mentorship is not merely a supplement to medical training but a foundational component of producing skilled, empathetic, and innovative physicians. This early guidance counters the often haphazard or passive exposure students receive in traditional curricula. The short-term objectives of the mentorship program focus on personalized academic and clinical support. These include:

- Providing structured and individualized guidance.
- Introducing diverse learning methodologies.
- Assisting mentees in preparing for hands-on clinical practice through simulation and observation.
- Equipping students with the tools necessary for success in competitive fields of medicine.

In parallel, the long-term goals of the Hoz Mentorship extend beyond knowledge transmission. They aim to support mentees in refining their surgical technique, cultivating leadership potential, enhancing personal growth, and establishing meaningful professional networks, both locally and internationally. The program fosters a culture of continuous improvement, where mentees are encouraged to give back by becoming future mentors themselves, thereby sustaining a cycle of excellence.

The Fundamental Values of the Mentorship

At the heart of the Hoz Neurosurgery Mentorship Program lies a firm commitment to the highest ethical, professional, and educational standards in medical training. One of the core tenets of the mentorship is active student engagement. Mentees are encouraged to participate meaningfully in shaping their learning experience through regular, structured feedback mechanisms, including anonymous surveys and one-on-one reflective sessions. This participatory approach reinforces mutual respect and accountability, allowing students to take ownership of their educational journey while also informing programmatic improvements.

Motivation and commitment to patient-centered care are regarded as non-negotiable entry criteria for mentees. Those invited into the mentorship are expected to display a sincere drive to learn, improve, and uphold the primacy of patient welfare. However, this motivation is not taken for granted, it is cultivated through a supportive environment that emphasizes personal growth, ethical responsibility, and clinical excellence.

Trust, in this context, is both a prerequisite and an outcome of the mentor–mentee relationship. It is built through unwavering transparency, honesty, and ethical conduct from both sides. No student is treated differently based on gender, background, age, or intellectual ability. Every mentee is treated with equal dignity, compassion, and respect, reflecting the mentorship's unwavering stance on equity and inclusivity.

The program also promotes a strong culture of teamwork and professional collaboration. Students are encouraged to work together on structured projects, case discussions, research initiatives, and peer-learning sessions. These interactions develop interpersonal competence and reinforce the importance of collective success in surgical practice. Conflict resolution strategies and structured training in respectful dialogue are also embedded in the mentorship, ensuring that communication remains constructive and emotionally intelligent even in high-pressure contexts.

Importantly, the program emphasizes personal responsibility. Mentees are held accountable for their actions, their influence on team dynamics, and their impact on patient care. By reinforcing the mentees' responsibility for their own progress, the program cultivates independence while sustaining mentorship as a protective and enabling force.

Ultimately, every medical student has the potential to become "a" doctor. But through value-driven mentorship, we aim to help them become "the" doctor. A physician defined not only by technical excellence but by character, compassion, and leadership.

Future Directions

Effective mentorship program is a critical part of the professional development of those engaged in medical careers. The main areas of program development scheme include accessibility of medical students to mentorship programs with more consideration for minority and underrepresented populations. Other areas represent the collaboration with policymakers to design high quality programs effectively and attempt to involve mentorship in the curriculum of medical education.

The integration of advanced technology within the training courses is achievable through the use of virtual reality, online sessions, and machine learning modalities. This can improve accessibility for students and time saving for both mentors and mentees. Moreover, creating a proper system of connections with stakeholders increases the chances of medical students finding top-grade opportunities in the research field and contributes to the growth of medical science from a young age. And finally, the program must have a safe environment to receive feedback and evaluation from the mentees through comprehensive tools. By applying these strategies, mentorship programs can evolve and be more effective in shaping the future of medical health professionals.

The current medical mentorship programs are committed to improving and adapting with different challenges. However, more research needs to be conducted to address the value, barriers, and outcomes of medical mentorship programs. The early guidance of medical students can have a favorable impact on the entire medical community and correspondingly on patient care. The sustainability of the mentor-mentee relationship is important to make healthcare professionals well-prepared, skilled, and supported when dealing with emergencies or complicated situations within the healthcare landscape.

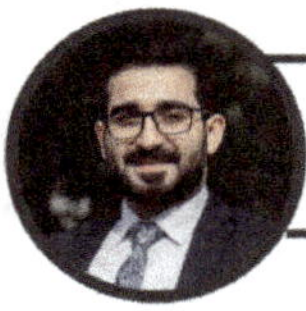

Aktham O. Al-Khafaji

s a fourth-year medical student, I found myself yearning for a deeper connection to the field of neurosurgery. My ascination with the brain had been there since my earliest days in medical school, and I had always envisioned yself as a surgically minded individual. But turning that passion into real-world experience had remained just out f reach. And to be honest, my earliest inspiration wasn't just academic—I owe a little of it to Dr. Derek Shepherd om ABC's *Grey's Anatomy*. Watching "McDreamy" in action planted the seed that being a brain surgeon was ot only brilliant, but also… cool. It may sound funny, but that spark mattered.

uring my second year of medical school, a literature review assignment led me to a YouTube video from Boston hildren's Hospital about Moyamoya disease—a rare cerebrovascular condition I had never heard of. The name trigued me, but it was the complexity of the disease that truly captivated me. The experience of studying this opic ignited a theoretical love for neurosurgery. Still, I longed for something beyond theory. I wanted to see eurosurgery in practice, to feel what it meant to be in that world. That chance finally came two years later when I as introduced to the Hoz Neurosurgery Mentorship Program by an acquaintance—who later became a very close iend. From the very beginning, the program offered far more than I expected. It wasn't just about shadowing eurosurgeons; it was about becoming part of something meaningful. It was my first real immersion into the world had only imagined.

he First Cut: An Unforgettable Sensory Experience: One of the most unforgettable moments came when I bserved my first neurosurgical procedure— evacuation of a subdural hematoma. The pungent, bitter smell of lectrocautery filled the OR. Most might find it unpleasant, but to me, it was intoxicating. It symbolized the alpable reality of the surgeries I had only read about. That scent marked the transition from theory to reality, from bserver to aspiring surgeon.

orging Bonds: The Strength of Teamwork: Another cornerstone of the mentorship was the emphasis on eamwork. We were held accountable not as individuals, but as a unit. Every success and every challenge was hared. This built a sense of solidarity that went beyond professional development—six years later, many of those entees remain among my closest friends.

rom Novice to Contributor: Embracing Research: Before the mentorship, I had no research experience—zero ublications, and little understanding of its role in medicine. Under the program's guidance, I came to appreciate ow research sharpens clinical thinking and broadens perspective. Today, I'm humbled to have co-authored over 0 publications, including articles and book chapters—something I never imagined when I first joined.

ull Circle: From Mentee to Resident: Six years later, as a neurosurgery resident, I look back at the Hoz lentorship Program as the foundation that made this all possible. It gave me not just skills and opportunities, but onfidence and clarity.

he Enduring Impact of Mentorship: The path to becoming a neurosurgeon is long and demanding—but entorship lights the way. The Hoz Neurosurgery Mentorship Program is more than a stepping stone; it's a ovement that has shaped many lives across Iraq and beyond. My journey, from curious student to committed esident, is proof of its power. And at the heart of it all is Dr. Hoz—a mentor whose belief in his students is ansformative. His vision built more than a mentorship program; it built a generation. No matter how far I go in is field, I'll always carry his influence with me.

References

1. Assael LA. Every surgeon needs mentors: a Halsteadian/Socratic model in the modern age. Journal of Oral and Maxillofacial Surgery. 2010 Jun 1;68(6):1217-8.
2. Barondess JA. Cushing and Osler: the evolution of a friendship. Transactions & Studies of the College of Physicians of Philadelphia. 1985 Jun 1;7(2):79-111.
3. Honavar SG. Mentoring is a serious business. Indian Journal of Ophthalmology. 2019 Dec 1;67(12):1915-7.
4. Zuckerman H. Scientific elite: Nobel laureates in the United States. Transaction Publishers; 1977.
5. Edelstein L. The Hippocratic Oath: text, translation and interpretation. Bulletin of the history of medicine/Supplements. 1943;1.
6. Gough I. Mentoring: historical origins and contemporary value. ANZ Journal of Surgery. 2008 Oct;78(10):831-.
7. Platz J, Hyman N. Mentorship. Clinics in colon and rectal surgery. 2013 Dec;26(04):218-23.
8. Newton I, Poster M. If I have seen further, it is only by standing on the shoulders of giants.
9. Souba WW. Mentoring young academic surgeons, our most precious asset. Journal of Surgical Research. 1999 Apr 1;82(2):113-20.
10. Obana KK, Obana WG. The Value of Medical Student Mentorship in Surgical Specialties. Hawai'i Journal of Health & Social Welfare. 2023 Jul;82(7):169.
11. ElHawary H, Salimi A, Gorgy A, Fesdekjian L, Seal A, Gilardino MS. Medical student mentorship in surgery: lessons learnt and future directions. Journal of Surgical Education. 2022 Jan 1;79(1):129-38.
12. Farkas AH, Allenbaugh J, Bonifacino E, Turner R, Corbelli JA. Mentorship of US medical students: a systematic review. Journal of general internal medicine. 2019 Nov;34:2602-9.
13. Caulfield M, Redden G, Sondheimer H. Graduation rates and attrition factors for US medical school students. AAMC Analysis in Brief. 2014;14(5).
14. Pinilla S, Nicolai L, Gradel M, Pander T, Fischer MR, von der Borch P, Dimitriadis K. Undergraduate medical students using Facebook as a peer-mentoring platform: a mixed-methods study. JMIR medical education. 2015 Oct 27;1(2):e5063.

15. Coates WC, Crooks K, Slavin SJ, Guiton G, Wilkerson L. Medical school curricular reform: fourth-year colleges improve access to career mentoring and overall satisfaction. Academic Medicine. 2008 Aug 1;83(8):754-60.
16. Sambunjak D, Straus SE, Marušić A. Mentoring in academic medicine: a systematic review. Jama. 2006 Sep 6;296(9):1103-15.
17. Maslow AH. A theory of human motivation. Psychological review. 1943 Jul;50(4):370.
18. Lam JA, Murray ER, Yu KE, Ramsey M, Nguyen TT, Mishra J, Martis B, Thomas ML, Lee EE. Neurobiology of loneliness: a systematic review. Neuropsychopharmacology. 2021 Oct;46(11):1873-87.
19. Hoz SS, Al-Sharshahi ZF, Aljuboori Z, Albanaa SA, Al-Awadi OM. The history and current status of neurosurgery in Iraq. World Neurosurgery. 2020 Aug 1;140:353-6.
20. Al-Khafaji AA, Hoz SS, Al-Awadi OM, Al-Sharshahi ZF. Alwitri: The father of modern neurosurgery in Iraq. Surgical Neurology International. 2021;12.

Section 1: Foundations of the Mentorship Program

CH.2: Designing the Hoz Neurosurgery Mentorship Infrastructure and Operational Framework

Rania H. Al-Taie, Fatima O. Ahmed, Zeena A. Alaaraji, Teeba A. Al-Ageely

Section 1: Foundations of the Mentorship Program

CH.2: Designing the Hoz Neurosurgery Mentorship Infrastructure and Operational Framework

A well-designed mentorship framework rests not only on defined roles, structured responsibilities, and organized administrative support, but on something far more human. Before delving into the operational details of the Hoz Neurosurgery Mentorship model, let us begin with the story of a student. A story that, perhaps, belongs to many of us.

He entered medical school with the noble intention of helping others. But beneath that lay deeper drivers curiosity, a hunger for knowledge, and a relentless pursuit of excellence. His passion for science was both his fuel and his burden. He was not boastful, nor was he overly academic in appearance. He held a deep, quiet respect for his professors, those who lifted him without diminishing others. For him, the study was not a task. It was meditation. He crafted learning strategies like an artisan, not merely to pass exams, but to be ready, truly ready, for scientific discourse and the responsibility of patient care.

Still, fear lingered. Fear of failure. Fear of an uncertain future. One question echoed from the first day of medical school: What will you do after graduation? He had known the answer for years, but lacked the courage to confront its implications. To protect himself, he chose solitude, controlling his journey with precision, walking alone because it felt safer.

But then, something shifted. His senior colleagues spoke about their transformative experiences with a mentorship. They shared how one mentor had reshaped not just their clinical skills, but their entire sense of purpose. Intrigued yet skeptical, the student quietly observed this mentor's work for almost a year, studying the trajectory, outcomes, and values embedded in the process. Only when convinced that this was more than hype did he apply, submitting a heartfelt motivation letter and a humble curriculum vita.

He never claimed to be the smartest applicant. But he knew one thing with certainty. No one would outwork him. Passion, even when it borders on self-inflicted pressure, was his defining trait.

The process began with online lectures and discussions, which were rigorous, challenging, and thought-provoking. He hadn't met the mentor in person yet. At times, the expectations encouraged him. At others, they overwhelmed him. Always preparing for the worst, he found it harder to prepare for the best.

Weeks later, he was selected to join in-person observerships in the operating room and emergency department. There, he met the mentor. A figure of resilience and calm. This mentor didn't dominate the room. He guided with discernment, knowing exactly when to push and when to step back. He listened to everyone. He noticed the details others missed. He trusted his mentees enough to let them lead in small but meaningful ways.

The student was quietly amazed. Not by theatrics, but by poise. And he realized something profound. Being ready for adversity is hard. But being ready for possibility is harder.

Time passed, and with it, growth. Surrounded by like-minded peers, generous residents, and seasoned consultants, the student's world expanded. Neurosurgery was no longer abstract. It was alive. An ecosystem of knowledge, collaboration, and mentorship. His career path crystallized. Ethical foundations were laid. Doors to training and research swung open.

But his hunger remained. Not for prestige, but for contribution. He wanted to give back, to create, to be part of the field's forward motion. His mentor affirmed that this was possible. He offered tools, introduced collaborators, and walked beside the student through research and discovery. The student's confidence grew. Not the dangerous kind, but the grounded confidence that safeguards patients and uplifts others. He became known. Professors noted him. Younger students sought his guidance. And with that recognition came responsibility. His mission had evolved. Not just to succeed, but to guide others toward clarity, purpose, and ethical action in medicine.

This student could be you. This mentor could be you. And this journey may already live within your story.

It is from this human foundation that the Hoz Mentorship Program was built. And it is through stories like this that we now turn to illustrate its structure.

Structuring the Hoz Mentorship Operations Team

Constructing a solid logistics team is crucial for program success. This segment explores the essential steps to create an outstanding team in the Hoz neurosurgery mentorship. The criteria to be included in the team is based on key elements like leadership skills, communication skills, and adaptation skills. Each team member must believe in the mutual aim and the vision of the mentorship. The team members must recognize the importance of continuous learning. The steps are as follows:

- **Strong baseline foundation:** building an excellent logistics team begins with setting a great leadership role model. The mentor must provide them with guidance and confidence in order to implant these abilities within each member. As a matter of fact, competent leaders steer the ship with finesse and be a source of inspiration for their coworkers and the mentees. They can provide guidance to ensure every mentee is on the same course of action and learning.
- **Clarifications of the tasks and responsibilities:** a well-organized team structure is key for its harmony. Detailed documentation of these information is essential to avoid any conflict or obstacle. The general roles of the logistic team involve registration of the student's information, timely and accurate delivery of learning materials to the students, managing collaborative events, coordinating and executing projects, implementing safety protocols for the students in the emergency room and operating rooms, well-documentations of the multifaceted aspects of the program, and expanding mentorship program by securing new projects and cooperation.
- **Effective communications:** members who communicate well speak with purpose, passion, and candor that permeates transparency throughout the program. An open flow of information is essential. It can be established through regular meetings, contact digital channels or other ways. Applying the practice of good communication would enhance contagious chemistry that can drive productivity.
- **The integration of advanced technology:** the implementation of technology can simplify tasks, improve efficiency, and ensure smooth workflow. The mentor and his team must remain up-to-date with the newest logistics software and tools. However, the integration of multiple new technologies can be stressful for the team. Challenges include compatibility issues, learning curves, and resistance to change need to be anticipated. Therefore, before introducing any new tool, make sure you understand its benefits to the team and evaluate the current situation or the problem you want to solve by using this tool. Once a mentor has decided to use it, a proper realistic and flexible plan about how to integrate the tool into the workflow need to be executed. A clear outlining of the integration steps, roles of the team, and the expected outcomes must be stated.

- **Continuous learning:** creating an exceptional team requires continuous improvement. The mentor should encourage the team to engage in learning and professional development opportunities in order to stay at the forefront of the program's needs. This requires dedication, meticulous planning, and a common vision.
- **Feedback and improvements:** well-constructed feedback is important. The Hoz mentorship provided an environment where team members could share feedback and offer their suggestions for refining strategies.

The facilitators' team is another important team that was constructed in the Hoz mentorship. This team is led by the mentor and includes doctors and graduated mentees. They played a vital role within the learning process of students. Their roles included supervision of clinical sessions, being a clinical course director or educational programs organizer. The essential duty of a medical facilitator is to elucidate the language of medical science to the learners' minds. Additionally, the facilitator is capable of empowering and the learner to grow as a competent doctor who is well-prepared to the challenges of the rapidly evolving health care world [1]. The main projects that was accomplished by the facilitators team include:

1. Online educational sessions about different topics including neuroanatomy, neuroradiology, neurosurgery case presentation, traumatic brain injury approach, intraoperative student etiquette and research training. In the virtual meeting, quizzes about the presented topics and differential diagnosis were performed. The students who give the correct answer have a better opportunity to attend the surgical operations.
2. Online interactive discussions that were mainly conducted by the mentor.
3. Hands-on physical trainings in suturing, microsuturing, burr hole drilling, aneurysmal clipping, micro-drilling, and imaging navigations. All were conducted on sheep animals and virtual reality models with the aid of UpSurgeon company [2]. Simulation plays a critical role in enhancing patient safety as it allows neurosurgical trainees to develop the requisite expertise [3-5].
4. A comprehensive overlap in the emergency room where students learned about the presentation, diagnosis, and management of many neurosurgical emergency cases like traumatic brain injury, intracranial hemorrhage, and neuro-oncological complications.
5. Guidance in the operating rooms and intensive care units in which the facilitator explains the indication, steps and follow-up plan of the surgery. Thus, the student becomes oriented

and capable of understanding the complex aspect of this complicated field. More precisely, the practical part of the mentorship involves two operative days per week. The mentees can attend neurovascular surgeries, tumors, and some diagnostic and therapeutic cerebral catheterizations. Safety measures included providing personal protective equipment that is mandatorily worn, requiring an official paper of complete COVID-19 vaccination for each participant. At the end of each surgery, the mentees had to stay and check on the patient's recovery and follow-up plan.

6. Training about the proper way of surgical scrubbing steps and benefits.
7. Addressing the main ethical considerations that must be acquired by the mentees on the levels of dealing with patients, communicating with the supervisor and working on research projects.
8. Accomplishing research projects that included case reports, clinical studies, review papers and books. In fact, every student who attended an operation is obligated to write a research paper or prepare a seminar presentation related to the details of the operation for the aim of educating medical students about research methodologies and neurosurgical perspectives.

The external representation team had the responsibility of executing meetings with national and international stakeholders. This team mainly consists of the mentor who sometimes invites students and doctors to observe and sometimes participate in the conversations. This initiative reflects the mentor's intentions to use every opportunity to teach his residents and mentees in scientific and practical levels. These meetings included the official agreement with the director of the neurosurgery teaching hospital, collaboration with the professors from Surgical Neurology International (SNI) journal, and participating in research projects with international doctors.

The other team is the advertisement team. They had the responsibility of documenting important moments in the mentorship through professional and illustrative images and videos. Then they create visionary announcements for the mentorship.

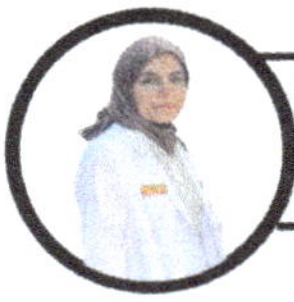

Zinah A. Alaraji

Unplanned paths often lead to the most extraordinary destinations. An unexpected encounter with Dr. Hoz had a profound impact on my life. This meeting was rooted in one of my life's most memorable and emotional experiences. I first saw Dr. Hoz at the Pan-Arab Dandy Neurosurgery Conference in Beirut, a city that holds deep, bittersweet significance for me. Having lost both of my parents there, Beirut became a place of immense pain, yet it also became the backdrop for one of the best "coincidences" of my life: meeting Dr. Hoz. His humility, warmth, and passion for teaching left an immediate impression on me. I realized that, in that city, I had gained a true mentor rather than losing someone once again.
At the conference, I learned about the Hoz Mentorship Program and its incredible work. Watching the students present their research and achievements was mesmerizing. It wasn't just me—everyone there was in awe of what they had accomplished under Dr. Hoz's guidance. It became clear to me that this program was not just about academics; it was about how a mentor like Dr. Hoz could bring out the best in his students, seeing potential in them even when no one else did. That was when I decided to get involved. Soon after, when the next mentorship cycle was about to start, Dr. Samer asked me to be one of the co-founders. It was one of the best—and scariest—decisions I've ever made. It became a transformative experience that fueled my passion for surgery and pushed me beyond my limits. Dr. Hoz's insights and approach sparked a shift in my focus, opening my eyes to new possibilities. I learned a great deal about neurosurgery up close by attending surgeries, shadowing neurosurgeons, meeting pioneers in the field, and working with the team on various research projects.

The Hoz Mentorship is not just about learning neurosurgery; it is about building a community where medicine unites us. We are more than colleagues—we are a family, connected by passion, curiosity, and a shared commitment to growth. Dr. Hoz's mentorship fosters an environment where everyone is valued for their potential, and together, we've created a bond rooted in science, compassion, and mutual respect. This bond, built on support and inspiration, defines what the Hoz Mentorship stands for: excellence, collaboration, and the belief that we rise higher when we lift each other.

Application Process and Criteria for Admission to the Hoz Mentorship Program

The students must apply for this course through an online form in which the mention their biographic and contact information then they upload a motivation letter and curriculum vitae. The form includes several questions that is designed for the aim of evaluating students' goals and expectations from the Hoz mentorship. Then, the application form is adjusted and reviewed by the mentor, who eventually selects the suitable students for this program after an online interview. The selection criteria included motivated students who have decided to apply for neurosurgery residency program after graduation or at least they're considering this option, it also includes young residents. The student must exhibit resilience and dedication. Extra points include good foundation in neuroscience, basic research skills and public health voluntary activities. The place of residency is important as the Hoz mentorship was established in Baghdad city, however, students from other cities are allowed to participate in both the online and practical training sessions. The mentorship included students from different stages of medical school.

Strategic Communication Framework

Effective communication is the backbone of any successful mentorship program. A well-structured communication plan defines the message, identifies the audience, sets the timing and channels, and establishes methods for tracking and feedback. In the long term, such planning significantly reduces miscommunication, saves time and resources, and ensures smooth program execution.

To streamline communication in the Hoz Neurosurgery Mentorship Program, a series of structured steps were adopted. First, we assessed existing strategies by evaluating communication outcomes with volunteers, funders, and partners. This audit helped us pinpoint what worked, what didn't, and where improvements were needed. The next step was identifying preferred communication channels, those most frequently used and most effective for our context.

Equally important was setting the cadence of communication. Frequency varies depending on audience type and platform, but consistency and clarity remained our priorities. We designated specific team members responsible for each communication task, ensuring accountability and timely delivery.

Crucially, documentation was emphasized. A communication plan is only as effective as its execution, and that requires detailed, shareable, and editable digital documentation. This transparency ensures that every team member and stakeholder operates with the same understanding, reducing ambiguity and enhancing collaboration. Our communication tools included:

- Zoom for virtual meetings held twice weekly
- Telegram for day-to-day messaging and coordination
- Official email for formal and academic correspondence

Additionally, in-person communication remained integral, particularly during clinical activities. Face-to-face interactions took place in hospital settings and the Hoz Lab, enabling real-time mentorship and feedback.

By integrating multiple platforms into a cohesive strategy, the program fostered a responsive, inclusive, and reliable communication environment.

Online Training in the Hoz Mentorship Program

A key pillar of the Hoz Neurosurgery Mentorship Program was a structured one-month online training course designed to provide foundational knowledge essential for neurosurgery. The curriculum included core topics such as neurosurgical anatomy, neuroimaging principles, the basics of operative techniques, and detailed analyses of neurosurgical procedural videography. These sessions laid the groundwork for clinical literacy and contextual understanding among mentees.

Zoom was the primary platform for delivering live interactive lectures and discussions, while Telegram served as a parallel channel for distributing written materials, collecting feedback, and facilitating asynchronous dialogue. The ease of access and user-friendliness of these platforms significantly increased engagement. Notably, participation in this virtual mentorship exceeded the combined enrollment of all seven previous in-person mentorship cycles, despite the concurrent challenges of the time, which made live sessions difficult to sustain.

The online format also expanded learning opportunities. Mentees engaged in public presentations about surgeries they observed or research projects they conducted, sharpening their academic communication and critical thinking skills. Furthermore, they participated in global discussions with neurosurgeons and academics from diverse countries, gaining valuable insights into international training pathways and innovations in the field.

By leveraging digital tools, the Hoz Mentorship not only maintained continuity during uncertain periods but also extended its reach, making high-quality neurosurgical education accessible to a broader, more diverse group of students. This model highlighted the potential of virtual training to democratize medical education and connect aspiring neurosurgeons with global thought leaders and emerging trends in the discipline.

Clinical Exposure in the Hoz Mentorship Program

The inception of modern neurosurgery in Iraq can be traced back to the 1970s. The developmental speed was somewhat modest, as indicated by the low number of neurosurgeons per population. Furthermore, there is a lack of enthusiasm among medical graduates in Iraq to pursue a career in neurosurgery due to the challenging nature of the job and the little rewards it offers. The user's text is enclosed in tags. Most medical schools primarily focus on neurosurgery during the senior years (5th and 6th year). In the early years of medical school, students are encouraged to independently explore the profession and pursue areas of interest. Consequently, the HOZ mentorship was established to facilitate the task and enhance accessibility to the field of neurosurgery. Moreover, it enhances the level of engagement among medical students in the field of neurosurgery through the establishment of a sequence of mentorship programs. Over the course of the last 6 years, the HOZ NeuroSurgery LAB in Neurosurgical Teaching Hospital, Baghdad, has organized eight mentorships. These mentorships have involved a total of 532 participants from various medical schools, aiming to offer students early experience to the field of neurosurgery. Selected students are allowed to participate in an observership period, during which they attend live lectures, seminars, and hands-on fundamental skills workshops. Furthermore, a primary goal for medical students in terms of clinical mentoring was to observe and learn from neurosurgery residents in various settings, such as the emergency department, operating room, and intensive care units. The user's text is enclosed in tags [6].

Beginning with clerkship lectures conducted over the course of a five-month period, the practical component of the mentorship was initiated. The students are able to attend neurovascular operations, tumors, and some diagnostic and therapeutic cerebral catheterizations on two of the seven days of the week that require them to undergo surgery. On each day of the surgery, there will be a maximum of four students permitted to attend the operation. Additionally, because of the extraordinary time period, the top goal was to ensure that the students were as safe as possible for the duration of the operation days. To do this, it was necessary to provide personal protection equipment that must be worn at all times, in addition to demanding an official document proving that each participant has received all of their vaccinations. Each time a patient underwent surgery, the trainees were required to remain and monitor their progress in recovery. In order to engage the greatest possible number of students simultaneously in various parts of neurosurgery, two students are present in the emergency department at the same time, and three students are present in the neurosurgical intensive care units. The feedback regarding the operation was collected at the end of each day. The students who attended the operation were asked to record their experiences, the lessons they learned, and even their sentiments throughout the procedure. These summaries were helpful, as they provided other students in the mentorship program with a better understanding of the protocol that should be followed in the operating room, the processes involved in the procedure, and the things that they should and should not do. In addition, after participating in a series of sessions designed to educate medical students about research, each of the four students who attended a surgery was required to submit a research paper that was connected to the operation in which they had participated.

HOZ Neurosurgery Lab

Microneurosurgery education and competence training are the primary focuses of the HOZ NeuroSurgery LAB, which is a facility managed by a team that is nonprofit. Dr. Samer S. Hoz, who was a senior neurosurgery resident at the time and is now a vascular neurosurgeon, established the aforementioned laboratory in June 2015. As a first step toward matching the neurosurgical training standards of developed countries, the Iraqi Association of Neurological Surgeons was initially in charge of supervising the laboratory. This facility can be found in Baghdad, specifically at the Neurosurgery Teaching Hospital. The principle that guides the lab's operations is "More Laboratory Simulation—Fewer Brain Complications." The ultimate purpose of this facility is to encourage residents' self-learning in a setting that is staff- and resource-constrained. This facility is probably the only facility of its kind in the country that is dedicated to neurosurgery trainees practicing and refining their skills in microscopic and vascular neurosurgery. Since that time, the laboratory has been recognized as a central location for surgical skills courses that have an emphasis on both fundamental and micro neurosurgery abilities. Residents are strongly encouraged to make use of the laboratory for the purpose of preoperative planning and training, as well as to hone essential neurosurgery skills like as suturing, bone work, and neurosurgical approach modeling through the utilization of animal-based and synthetic training models. Particular emphasis is placed on microneurosurgical procedures, which include hand movements under the microscope, the implantation of micro-sutures, and the atraumatic manipulation of a variety of tissues. In order to achieve the goal, it is necessary to sustain ongoing training, not necessarily for a particular operation, but rather for an expanding variety of approaches.

When Professor Franco Servadi, President of the World Federation of Neurosurgical Societies (WFNS), presented the laboratory as a "good example of education from the perspective of global neurosurgery" at the World Federation of Neurosurgical Societies Symposium in 2018, a significant milestone was reached in the journey of the laboratory where it is currently located [7]. The main goal of the lab was to accomplish the following:

- Demonstrate a paradigm for the development of neurosurgical abilities in settings with limited resources.
- Challenge the culture that is currently in place by highlighting simulation as a beneficial tool for improving patient outcomes.
- Encourage residents to complete their education and expand their skills.
- Provide residents with a learning environment that is both independent and easy to access.
- Prompt medical students and residents to seek careers in research by providing encouragement.
- Give neurosurgeons the opportunity to continue cultivating their skills.

The laboratory consists of a solitary room of 4 - 6 meters, which is further separated into three separate stations. The first station is equipped with a cost-effective microscope that is installed on a table. The microscope has a maximum magnification of 20x and is coupled to a high-definition camera. The camera is combined with a display screen. The two remaining stations consist of surgical loupes (4.3 surgical loupes equipped with LED lights) for practicing fundamental suturing procedures and operating approaches. This setup allows the trainee to practice and understand the usefulness of these two surgical instruments while doing different duties. Furthermore, the laboratory is furnished with a versatile orthodontic drill capable of accommodating different types and sizes of burrs. It also contains sutures, a custom-made micro suturing pad, an anastomosis training kit consisting of silastic tubes, a double-clamp vascular clip, and a patency tester. Additionally, there is a collection of used instruments, such as burrs, suction devices, mono-bi-polar coagulation devices, and microinstruments. Simulations commonly utilize locally sourced, readily available animal-based training specimens, such as chicken or turkey feet and wings, as well as fresh heads of sheep and cow models. The lab's accomplishments and main results from its beginning until now are as follows:

- Established the inaugural structured neurosurgery department in the nation.

- Organized and facilitated 53 sessions focused on developing abilities in micro-neurosurgery, encompassing techniques such as micro-suturing, vascular micro-neurosurgery, micro-drilling, and modeling different cranial approaches.
- Organized eight elective rotation cycles for medical students, involving a total of 532 participants.
- Pioneered the creation of the initial integrated research unit, resulting in over 70 published works to date.

Although there is ample evidence supporting the effectiveness of simulation as a valuable training method in neurosurgery, especially in microneurosurgery, the availability of simulation and training opportunities is restricted in low- and middle-income countries (LMICs) due to various reasons, most of which cannot be easily resolved in the near future. We have showcased how our expertise has transformed the provision of medical treatment for patients and facilitated the establishment of a previously nonexistent specialized field in cerebrovascular surgery inside the country. Furthermore, although simulation has not yet been officially incorporated into neurosurgery training programs in most LMICs, it has the potential to be a helpful tool for enhancing training consistency and standardizing assessment processes.

Evaluations and Feedback in the Hoz Mentorship Program

Feedback is crucial for efficient communication since it allows the provider to verify if their message has been comprehended and received as intended and make adjustments to their communication approach if necessary. It also plays a vital role in facilitating effective two-way communication by promoting mutual understanding and minimizing the risk of misinterpretation or ambiguity. Additionally, it enhances the connections of trust and rapport between the giver and the recipient. Providing constructive feedback on communication is an essential characteristic of effective leadership. It facilitates the support of each team member in improving their ability to communicate with their colleagues, students, and stakeholders and express their needs and concerns. Feedback can be provided through speaking or nonverbal communication, written remarks, facial expressions, or body language. Although negative feedback can be employed to identify areas for improvement, positive feedback is often used to bolster and motivate good communication. The sorts of feedback include formal feedback that follows a straightforward and objective format. This allows both the doctor and mentees to discuss areas of improvement in their work and communication strategy. Prescriptive feedback is a type of guidance where the mentees inform the mentor on how to improve their work methods.

The Effectiveness of the Hoz Mentorship Program

In a previous study that we conducted to assess the effectiveness of the neurosurgical mentorship program during its ninth Hoz neurosurgery mentorship program, we observed that exposure to neurosurgery had increased the generally positive impressions regarding the specialty of neurosurgery, which was reflected through the improvement of the academic and curricular potential of medical students in neurology and neurosurgery using surveys for the assessment and comparison of the pre-course and post-course survey. The results of this study illustrated an observable improvement in neurosurgical knowledge with over 5% increase in the rate of passing scores in only 1 month. It also resulted in the development of the research experience and interest as multiple research teams were formed following the course, which contributed to the growing academic productivity of the participants. The personal progress among participants was also a prominent outcome, as experiences are different, participants shared their feedback at the end of the course, highlighting the most advantages they gained during the short span of a month [8].

The self-funded, diverse, and widely inclusive nature of the program emphasized the importance of educational programs and mentor-mentee relationships. With a focus on empathy, teamwork, and leadership, the program fostered personal and professional growth, setting a standard for future initiatives that share similar aims and objectives [8].

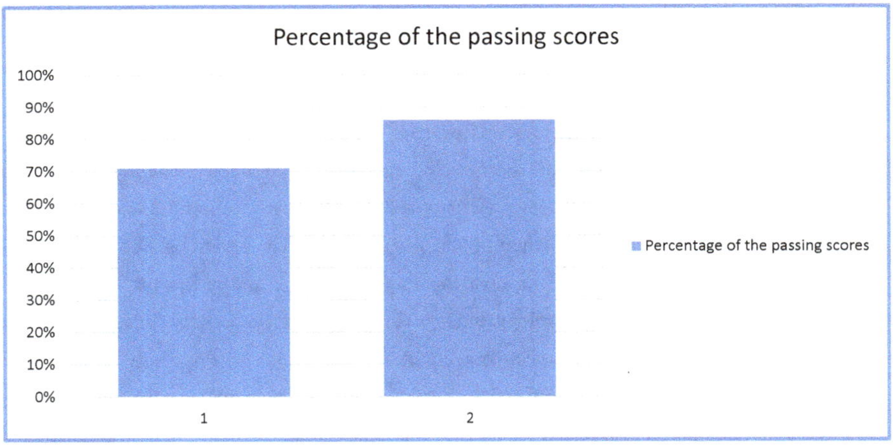

Figure 1: Chart showing the improvement in the passing rate in pre-mentorship scores (1), and post-mentorship scores (2).

References

1. NAWAZ S, RAZAQ N, SARFRAZ F, SARFRAZ F, ULLAH MS, MASOOD A. Perception of Faculty of their Role as Medical Facilitator. Pakistan Journal of Medical and Health Sciences. 2021;15(11):3337-9.
2. https://www.upsurgeon.com/
3. Konakondla S, Fong R, Schirmer CM. Simulation training in neurosurgery: advances in education and practice. Adv Med Educ Pract. 2017;8:465–73. 4.
4. Akhtar KS, Chen A, Standfield NJ, Gupte CM. The role of simulation in developing surgical skills. Curr Rev Musculoskelet Med. 2014;7(2):155–60. 5.
5. Coelho G, Zanon N, Warf B. The role of simulation in neurosurgery. Childs Nerv Syst. 2014;30(12):1997–2000.
6. Hoz SS, Ismail M, Almufadhal MH, Al-Ageely TA, Aljuboori Z. Reinvigorating medical student mentorships in neurosurgery during the pandemic: Lessons learned from Iraq. Surgical Neurology International. 2022;13.
7. WFNS. WFNS Symposia 2018eKuala Lumpur, Malaysia|WFNS. Available at: https://www.wfns.org/newsletter/44. Accessed June 20, 2021.
8. Al-Ageely TA, Ismail M, Al-Araji ZA, Abdulsada AM, Algburi HA, Akar NM, Hoz SS. Effectiveness of mentorships and early exposure in Neurosurgery. World Neurosurgery. 2023 Oct 1;178:e773-6.

Section 1: Foundations of the Mentorship Program

CH.3: Ensuring Hoz Mentorship Program Sustainability in Low-Resource Neurosurgical Settings

Rania H. Al-Taie, Jaafer AbdulWahid, Mohammed A. Al-Dhahir, Teeba A. Al-Ageely

Section 1: Foundations of the Mentorship Program

CH.3: Ensuring Hoz Mentorship Program Sustainability in Low-Resource Neurosurgical Settings

The support and promotion of advancements and learning opportunities for medical students and junior neurosurgeons is a major factor in the significance of mentorships in medical education and neurosurgery. Organizing a mentoring program in accordance with the intended audience offers to fulfill various interests and improve education. One of the primary problems with the majority of programs that have already been put into place is their sustainability and incapacity to sustain ongoing mentorship cycles. This has a detrimental effect and has resulted in an interrupted learning pattern, which eventually causes participants' engagement and interest to wane. This issue is particularly noticeable in war-torn nations like Iraq when outside factors cause the educational process to stall and the resources needed for such initiatives and training sessions to run out. Especially in wide and complex fields like neurosurgery, an effective way to foster learning and promote advancement is through an adequately supported long-term mentorship program. Furthermore, the primary aims are providing direction and therapy to assist the mentees in achieving their future aspirations [1,2]. Even though these programs are regarded as a necessary and fundamental component of medical education, they are seen as a luxury in places with little funding and a lack of mentors and providers, especially in war-torn nations like Iraq, where it is very difficult to find and maintain these kinds of programs. Additionally, developing and executing mentorship programs may present chances to enhance, encourage, and maintain the educational and learning process for students, enhancing their academic performance and offering guidance and a forward-looking perspective to those just starting their medical careers [3].

Challenges to Sustain a Medical Mentorship

There are very few educational programs overall and mentorship programs specifically focused on neurosurgery, and their duration is only brief due to a variety of factors, including low participation rates, a lack of interest, and inadequate program planning. Furthermore, with the establishment of the first tertiary neurosurgery hospital (Neurosurgery Teaching Hospital) in the nation's capital, Baghdad, in 1972, the first official neurosurgical training pathway in Iraq was formed relatively recently. Since then, only a small number of further specialized facilities have been built in Baghdad and a few other areas of Iraq. Additionally, there have been no policy changes for further advancement in this specialization, and the majority of attempts to develop it in Iraq have been individual ones [4,5]. However, many mentorship programs that have been put into place struggle to remain sustainable over several cycles, particularly in the field of neurosurgery. This is particularly noticeable in countries plagued by conflict where there are barriers and diverting events that center on these kinds of activities.

Surgical mentorship programs in low-resource environments face several significant sustainability challenges, which hinder their effectiveness and long-term impact. One of the foremost obstacles is resistance to change. Many healthcare providers, particularly senior surgeons, may be reluctant to adopt new techniques introduced through mentorship. This resistance stems from the comfort and familiarity with established routines, which can lead to a reluctance to embrace innovative surgical methods. Such resistance can create barriers to the adoption of new skills and diminish the overall efficacy of mentorship programs. Another critical challenge is the limitation of resources. Most low-resource settings have a serious shortage of experienced surgical mentors, along with an inability to maintain access to recent surgical equipment and sterile environments. These shortages are critically hindering the capacity for effective mentorship, whereby both mentors and mentees are struggling with outdated tools and techniques. For that matter, unless the right resources are in place, transferring knowledge and skills will be difficult, and the quality of training will be at jeopardy. Financial constraints also pose a significant threat to the sustainability of surgical mentorship programs. Adequate funding is essential to cover the costs of mentor recruitment, training, and operational support. However, many low-resource settings struggle to secure the necessary financial resources. This lack of funding often leads to suboptimal mentor compensation, which in turn causes reluctance among experienced professionals to participate in these programs. Additionally, limited departmental budgets further constrain investments in mentorship initiatives, preventing their growth and sustainability [6].

Logistical and Technological Challenges: In most resource-limited settings, geographic dispersion and lack of infrastructure hamper effective interactions for mentorship. Internet connectivity is patchy, interfering with virtual mentorship opportunities that can bridge the gap between mentors and mentees across distances. Besides, the need for actual physical travel to very distant places contributes to the logistics complexities: poor transport infrastructure interferes with timely and regular mentoring [6].

Last but not least, the time factor represents a significant issue in the optimization of surgical mentorship programs. Mentors are generally overwhelmed by clinical work in low-resource settings and thus can devote very limited time to mentoring trainees. This then brings up inadequate interaction between the mentor and mentees at the cost of compromising the depth in the training experience. Besides that, the limited time of mentorship visits, coupled with fluctuations in cases of patients, might also further limit exposure to surgery skills training and detract from the effectiveness of such programs.

In their evaluation of a mentoring program for junior medical staff at a pediatric hospital, Stewart et al. (2023) [7] emphasized several difficulties regarding sustainability. The long-term relationships found it hard to be sustained beyond the time of the formal mentoring program. While many mentors and mentees continued their interactions, the practical constraints of distance and the pressure of busy schedules made it hard to sustain these contacts. Moreover, the program was set to be on a voluntary basis; it, therefore, does not guarantee regular engagement for both parties. According to Stewart et al., such initiatives take time to develop and thus require continuous institutional support and resources to allow the initiative to remain sustainable over time.

These are some of the sustainability challenges that require innovative strategies on how virtual mentorship platforms can be integrated, sustainable funding models developed, and supportive policies created in order to promote long-term mentorship engagement.

Hoz Mentorship Sustainability Framework

The primary problem with a wide range of extracurricular medical education programs is that they are inconsistent, which disrupts the learning process and may eventually make participants lose interest in the program altogether. One potential issue with sustainability could be the recurrence of materials and contents in these kinds of initiatives. Without a doubt, medical education is an ongoing process with no clear conclusion. Therefore, over time, relevant material, improved knowledge acquired, and an inclination in interests are produced by the consistency and renewability of programs like mentorships.

Our experience has shown that, despite the unique circumstances and scarce resources, running a neurosurgery mentoring program nine times over the previous six years in a conflict zone like Iraq has resulted in a good understanding of the significance of educational continuity. We were successful in recruiting 1116 participants for our neurosurgery mentorship programs over the course of its nine cycles. Most of these participants were medical students who were considering neurosurgery as a potential career path. Additionally, postgraduates and neurosurgery residents were included in the mentorship. Iraq makes up 90% of the recruiting pool overall, with the remaining 10% coming from 17 other nations. The lack of easily available information opened up creative possibilities for developing fresh approaches to instruction and altered training regimens. The following strategies were implemented by us to guarantee a sustainable framework:

- Regarding the subjects covered throughout each mentoring cycle, there were no set or repeated timetables. This was done in an effort to guarantee originality and the distinct experience of every batch.
- The subjects were chosen with the great majority of students, residents, and specialists in mind in order to best suit their needs and captivate their interests. Therefore, the topics would include everything from exact neurosurgical features and operative views to basic anatomy orientation.
- There was a discussion of a number of clinically relevant subjects, including neuro-oncology, neurophysiology, traumatic brain injury, cerebrovascular surgery, and critical care.
- Dr. Samer S. Hoz, a senior neurosurgeon with extensive experience in medical education, research, and the neurosurgical field, led the program. As such, clinical research and medical writing skills were essential components of each cycle, giving participants the knowledge they needed to begin contributing to numerous research papers.
- Through the use of an online platform, numerous neurosurgeons with a variety of specializations from all over the world were invited to participate by giving presentations detailing their experiences choosing to specialize in neurosurgery as a career, providing in-depth analyses of various neurosurgical subspecialties and going over the many therapeutic options used in neurosurgery. Additionally, a few residents presented talks to share their perspectives on neurosurgery training and residency as well as their personal experiences.

- Surgical training skills additionally served a significant part in several cycles. Regardless of the participants' academic levels, the mentorship also featured case discussions, which played a significant role in the program's training process due to the numerous clinical, theoretical, and ethical components that are linked with them.
- The main objective of this mentorship program is to give medical students and residents information about the sector that is being considered as a potential career path so that they may make better decisions in the future. It's crucial to remember that even with the significant increase in neurosurgical knowledge, participants still need to complete enough clinical training to be eligible for residency.
- When applying to mentorship programs, mentees have a variety of options to choose from. In our nine neurosurgery mentorship program, we discovered that the majority of candidates' primary objective is to observe the issues out of interest; early-stage medical students make up the majority of this category. This can be partially explained by the fact that medical students primarily look to mentorship programs in medical education as an extracurricular enrichment to improve their academic performance. It's also crucial to remember that a large number of participating students apply, wherever possible, to programs that are associated with other areas of interest. The desire to receive mentorship during their medical education and specialization orientation is another prevalent motive for applying. Other motivations include the desire to learn more about the field of neurosurgery and advance one's knowledge and experience, the goal of enhancing one's resume through involvement in mentor-provided activities like research enrollment, and the desire to network, which is particularly strong in mentorship programs that meet international standards. Understanding this aspect is crucial to implementing suitable strategies to ensure sustainability.
- In modern mentorship programs, technology is leveraged to make access and addressing of concerns much easier. Virtual mentorship hubs make it possible for mentors and mentees to connect through telemedicine tools across distances that have been shrunk by geographical boundaries. These further allow for real-time interactions, with continued support from a mentorship that is independent of physical locations. Besides, it's quite easy to set up online resource libraries where mentees can use their time most valuably in educational respects, enabling them to study at their own pace and retain the information

better. By engaging these technological solutions, mentorship programs may more easily be sustained and adapt to a constantly evolving medical landscape.

- Engagement of mentees is very important with regard to the success of mentorship programs. The establishment of mechanisms for regular feedback enables organizers to understand their needs and continually work on enhancing effectiveness. Such feedback is intended to find out problems, modify strategies taken to date, and keep relevant activities pursued with regard to the goals that mentees are seeking to achieve. In addition, customized matching through algorithms or questionnaires enhances the pairing of mentors with mentees. Personalized matching considers personal interests, career goals, and even communication styles to provide a more productive relationship that will be tailor-fit and meaningful.
- Institutionalization gives the frameworks for sustaining mentorship programs. Embedding mentorship within institutions through policies and curricula makes the process formal and, hence, core to the institution's culture. This makes sure people do not consider mentorship an optional activity but rather an integral component of professional development. Leadership support is equally important; the active championing of the program on the part of senior leadership and key stakeholders' nets commitment that inspires participation within the organization. It helps ensure valuable resources are available, instills a sense of accountability, and raises the profile of the program across the organization.

Our mentoring program's primary target audience was medical students, but it also included a variety of subjects that may captivate the interest of senior interns, residents, and doctors at the same time. These planning techniques can provide a clear direction for the mentorship program and its intended audience. They can also strengthen the mutually beneficial relationship between mentors and mentees by emphasizing the mentees' interests, abilities, and aspirations. This experience also lays the groundwork for continuing and upcoming employed programs, which might benefit immensely from growing into partnerships with other local institutions that can offer neurosurgical orientation as well as enhanced surgical training skills. International cooperation may also be very beneficial for conferences, recognizing the benefits of networking, and providing possibilities for more advanced training.

Building on Existing Knowledge for Future Innovation

In this section, we delve into existing research and theoretical frameworks surrounding mentorship in medical education. This comprehensive review aims to synthesize key findings from previous studies, highlighting effective strategies, challenges, and outcomes associated with mentorship programs across diverse medical disciplines. By examining the evolution of mentorship models and their impact on professional development, this section establishes a scholarly foundation that informs the sustainability and efficacy of mentorship in enhancing medical training. This exploration not only underscores the importance of structured mentorship in medical education—a topic crucial for fostering future healthcare leaders—but also aligns with ongoing efforts to elevate educational standards.

Caruso et al. (2019) [8] present findings from multiple Graduate Medical Education (GME) training programs on the sustainability of mentorship programs. They implemented a five-step mentorship model in an effort to increase match rates through an emphasis on frequent mentor-mentee interactions and self-selection. Results showed that mentorship relationships were established and, more importantly, were persevered over time, as evidenced by the considerable rise in both the number and usefulness of mentor relationships. This was furthered by structured, ongoing meetings for sustainability and the flexibility for mentees to select mentors based on mutual interests. Geesa et al. (2022) [9], in their study, raise concern for fluidity in the sustainability of the mentorship program design to meet emerging needs. Indeed, the authors identified that a sustainable mentorship program should move toward meeting academic and professional needs. For this, continuous feedback from its stakeholders is very necessary. Increased flexible modes of delivery and networking opportunities are needed. Essentially, be aligned with the progress of the mentees and thus their readiness for the program, to ensure success in the long run and to make sure that mentors and mentees will continue to be engaged.

In their paper on group mentorship programs for undergraduate medical students, Skjevik et al. (2020) [10] discuss several sustainability challenges that arise in medical education mentorship initiatives. They emphasize that group mentorship programs, while beneficial, often face difficulties such as ensuring consistent participation and balancing mentor workloads. Additionally, the financial and time investments required for long-term programs can create obstacles to their sustainability. To address these challenges, Skjevik et al. suggest integrating mentorship more thoroughly into the medical school curriculum and providing institutional support for both mentors and mentees.

Straus et al. (2008) [11], in their work toward the development of a mentorship strategy, identify several key challenges to sustainability within mentorship programs in academia. According to them, there is a realization that mentorship in academic medicine is central to career development; however, several impediments may greatly contrast the sustainability of such programs. These are increased clinical, research, and administrative loads among mentors, lack of formal mentorship systems, and lack of recognition of mentorship efforts by academic institutions. It is inferred that mentorship programs should be codified with training events for both mentors and mentees and with institutional support for mentorship activities as a means of enhancing sustainability.

The paper by Balandya et al. (2021) [12] highlights some of the key sustainability issues in research mentoring programs in resource-limited settings. Notably, the authors emphasize that for building research capacity, there is a need for both vertical and peer-to-peer mentorship approaches. On the other hand, limiting factors identified include limited funding for research, lack of protected time to conduct research, and irregular engagement in mentorship due to competing priorities. According to Balandya et al., enhancing the sustainability of efforts like the creation of collaborative environments, structured research training, and the inclusion of mentorship across academic hierarchies will assist in longitudinal development in research.

The core of the innovative mentorship behavior model by Hussain et al. (2021) [13] within higher education mentorship programs is the sustainability concept. They make it crystal clear that mentorship would become full-blown and even sustainable when it addresses the key factors of career support, intellectual growth, psychosocial development, and research supervision. In this regard, the investigation draws the final statements on the nature of the mentorship process: it is or has to be relentlessly in the development phase to generate benefits for both parties, that is, mentors and mentees. As such, Hussain et al. call for the necessity of organized mentorship programs supported by institutional policies that help in long-term academic and professional development.

In medical education, mentorship programs play a crucial role in providing students and residents with early exposure to their chosen specialty. This can be difficult in low-income nations or in unique situations where programs' sustainability is significantly impacted, like conflict zones. The reliance and sustainability of such initiatives are significantly increased by designing and evaluating the mentorships' vision and objectives primarily based on the experiences of the mentors and the participants. To determine the actual costs, benefits, and institutional effects of mentorship programs, a formal, long-term evaluation of their effectiveness is required. Changes toward pro-mentorship cultures have the potential to significantly enhance medical results and happiness for both individuals and institutions. There is still much to learn about the mentoring process, especially in light of theories that contend that each stakeholder's impact and function are interwoven and call for close examination.

Our concept of mentorship aims to go beyond current notions in order to provide more direction for the design and management of mentoring programs and to identify important areas for urgently needed future study.

References

1. Caruso TJ, Steinberg DH, Piro N, Walker K, Blankenburg R, Rassbach C, Marquez JL, Katznelson L, Dohn A. A strategic approach to implementation of medical mentorship programs. J Grad Med Educ. 2016;8(1):68–73.
2. Clutterbuck D. Everyone needs a mentor- Fostering talent in your organization. 5th ed. London: CIPD; 2014
3. Kurré J, Bullinger M, Petersen-Ewert C, Guse AH. Diferential mentorship for medical students: development, implementation and initial evaluation. Int J Med Educ. 2012;1:3.
4. Faraj MK. Are innovation and creativity possible in a country at war? My story of neurosurgery in Baghdad, Iraq. Surg Neurol Int. 2022;13:402. 5.
5. Hoz SS, Al-Sharshahi ZF, Aljuboori Z, Albanaa SA, Al-Awadi OM. The history and current status of neurosurgery in Iraq. World Neurosurgery. 2020;1(140):353–6.
6. Awuah WA, Tan JK, Bharadwaj HR, Aderinto N, Ferreira T, Patel H, Shah MH, Kapoor AA, Banerjee S, Abdul-Rahman T, Atallah O. Surgical mentorship in low-resource environments: Opportunities and challenges, a perspective. Health Science Reports. 2024 Aug;7(8):e2258.
7. Stewart B, Polley C, Gray A. Evaluation of a mentoring program for junior medical staff at a tertiary paediatric hospital: Uptake, impact and sustainability. Focus on Health Professional Education: A Multi-Professional Journal. 2023 Sep 1;24(3):47-60.
8. Caruso TJ, Kung T, Piro N, Li J, Katznelson L, Dohn A. A sustainable and effective mentorship model for graduate medical education programs. Journal of graduate medical education. 2019 Apr 1;11(2):221-5.
9. Geesa RL, McConnell KR, Brown RD. Mentorship for doctor of education candidates: Exploring sustainability, networking, and expected outcomes within a mentoring program. Journal of Research on Leadership Education. 2022 Sep;17(3):291-309.
10. Skjevik EP, Boudreau JD, Ringberg U, Schei E, Stenfors T, Kvernenes M, Ofstad EH. Group mentorship for undergraduate medical students—a systematic review. Perspectives on medical education. 2020 Oct;9:272-80.

11. Straus SE, Graham ID, Taylor M, Lockyer J. Development of a mentorship strategy: a knowledge translation case study. Journal of continuing education in the health professions 2008 Jun;28(3):117-22.

12. Balandya E, Sunguya B, Gunda DW, Kidenya B, Nyamhanga T, Minja IK, Mahande M, Mmbaga BT, Mshana SE, Mteta K, Bartlett J. Building sustainable research capacity at higher learning institutions in Tanzania through mentoring of the Young Research Peers. BMC medical education. 2021 Dec;21:1-1.

13. Hussain S, Tirmizi SM, Mutahir H. An Innovative Mentorship Behavior Model Imperative for Sustainable Higher Education. Int. J. Innov. Creat. Change. 2021;15:335-49.

14. Al-Ageely TA, Ismail M, Alaraji ZA, Abdulwahid J, Ayad F, Jaafar H, Aktham A, Salih HR, Hoz S. Planning a sustainable neurosurgery mentorship program in a war-torn country: experience from Iraq. Chinese Neurosurgical Journal. 2024 Aug 2;10(1):23.

Section 1: Foundations of the Mentorship Program

CH.4: Creating a Structured Curriculum for Neurosurgical Education and Skill Development

Rania H. Al-Taie, Sama Albairamani, Mustafa Ayad Murayati, Teeba A. Al-Ageely

Section 1: Foundations of the Mentorship Program

CH.4: Creating a Structured Curriculum for Neurosurgical Education and Skill Development

Simulation is an instructional technique in which a learner can engage in a real-life activity in a virtual environment that is safe and controlled. It serves a crucial role in the training of neurosurgeons, enabling them to acquire the necessary skills to improve patient safety [1]. Neurosurgical simulation has utilized a diverse array of materials, both biological and non-biological. These materials include live animals, cadavers, synthetic models, and computer-based models. When compared to non-biological materials, the utilization of nonliving animals offers several additional benefits, such as cost-effectiveness, resemblance to human anatomy, immediate haptic feedback, and easy accessibility [2].

Neurosurgery is a highly diverse discipline that necessitates an advanced understanding of anatomy and exceptional technical accuracy. This pressing requirement necessitates a swift augmentation of the worldwide neurosurgical workforce, particularly in LMICs. Regrettably, those nations are experiencing resource shortages as a result of social disparities and economic limitations. In light of this context, a study conducted by the World Federation of Neurological Societies (WFNS) found that 26.8% of LMICs reported insufficient availability of necessary neurosurgical equipment [3].

Neurosurgery is a delicate specialty that requires intricate skills and knowledge. Early exposure to such skills is highly encouraged to make individuals more oriented and precise. Significant development has been made in the simulation of vascular, particularly endovascular and neurosurgery. The complexity and variability of cranial procedures make simulation challenging, but significant progress has been made recently [4].

Cadaver-Free Simulation Training in Microneurosurgery

Traditionally, the majority of neurosurgery training occurred within the confines of the operating room, where residents acquired practical skills by assisting in a multitude of surgical procedures. Nevertheless, several problems need to be addressed to provide effective training. These challenges include the need for a sufficient number of cases, the importance of maintaining efficiency during surgery, constraints on resident work hours, and a greater focus on patient safety and outcome measurements. As a result, there have been efforts to find suitable additional training methods. The challenges in cranial microneurosurgical training are intensified by the extended duration of operations, the limited space for operating, and the need for further training in skills such as hand-eye coordination, visual feedback, precise manipulation, and control of physiological tremors. While cadaveric courses have long been a crucial component of neurosurgical training, their inherent limitations have prompted intensive efforts to create more practical alternatives that tackle issues such as cost, accessibility, and the need for human resource investment. These challenges are particularly burdensome in LMICs. The development of low-cost, skill-based simulation training systems has been driven by recent developments in digital interfaces, improved availability of mobile technology, and a growing interest in enhancing global neurosurgical training standards [5].

However, there is a lack of literature regarding the inclusion and implementation of these techniques in formal neurosurgical training programs, as well as their immediate and long-term effects. The possibility of offering these courses in a setting with low resources has shown that such experiences have the capacity to promote education in neurosurgery in economically disadvantaged countries [6].

Cadaver-Free Simulation Training in Hoz Mentorship

A simulation course, which did not involve the use of cadavers, was implemented at the Neurosurgery Teaching Hospital in Baghdad, Iraq. This course was conducted as a part of a global training project that was supported by the World Federation of Neurosurgical Societies. The purpose of the course was to showcase the practicality of implementing a bigger-scale application in other LMICs. The course platform was specifically developed to facilitate psychomotor training in microneurosurgery. It incorporates virtual reality to enhance mental training, mixed reality to assist with hybrid training, and physical reality to promote manual training. The duration of the course was 2 days, amounting to a total of 8 hours. The individuals who were invited included attending neurosurgeons, senior neurosurgery residents (with 3 to 6 years of experience), junior neurosurgery residents (with 1 to 2 years of experience), and medical students. Prior to the course, a train-the-trainer session was conducted to familiarize teachers with the concept of hybrid simulation training, the operation of the simulators, and the specific duties that each participant is expected to perform. A total of six hyperrealistic neurosurgical simulators were utilized during the training. These simulators were generously given by UpSurgeOn, in a nonprofit project. The simulators were created to instruct in surgical microneuroanatomy, specifically the pterional, subtemporal, and retrosigmoid approaches, as well as techniques for treating common brain aneurysms. These techniques include clipping the internal carotid artery bifurcation, anterior communicating artery, middle cerebral artery bifurcation, posterior communicating artery, and basilar tip aneurysms. The practical session started with cognitive training using the neuroanatomy and head atlas setup (mobile application), advanced to a combination of training using hybrid neuroanatomy and craniotomy planning (augmented reality), and ended with hands-on training in craniotomy and dura opening. The training program emphasized the cultivation of both cognitive and physical abilities. Automatization, inventiveness, and strategy exemplify cognitive abilities, whereas dexterity and quickness exemplify physical abilities. Every participant moved in a consecutive manner through the 5 main stations. The initial two focused on cognitive ability, while the remaining three stressed practical skills and as follows:

- Station 1: focuses on microneuroanatomy, aims to stimulate the learner's creativity by utilizing a realistic anatomical brain model and its corresponding mobile application.
- Station 2: known as hybrid planning, focused on the precise placement of the patient, strategizing the incision, and carefully choosing the target.
- Station 3: the medical procedure craniotomy was taught through hands-on instruction utilizing a disposable skull set. A total of 18 craniotomies were done.
- Station 4: also known as microexploration, was specifically created to introduce the participants to the typical neurovascular structures and allow them to gain hands-on experience in performing microsurgical aneurysm cutting. The main objectives of this station were to acquaint participants with the surgical loupe, microscope, and endoscope. Additionally, it aimed to help participants gain a comprehension of the coordination between the eyes, hands, and feet that is necessary when using the surgical microscope. It also provided participants with an opportunity to practice the angulation techniques employed with the endoscope, as well as the manipulation limits and identifiable anatomical structures.
- Station 5: it consisted of instruction on the dura and the skin closure techniques.

The course had a total of thirty trainees, consisting of six attending neurosurgeons, seven senior-level residents, nine junior-level residents, and eight medical students. Trainee response following the course was evaluated using a 5-point Likert scale. The overall experience was highly rated, with an average of 98% of respondents indicating agreement or strong agreement to questions evaluating the course's value based on metrics such as surgical orientation, anatomical accuracy of the models, tactile feedback during manipulation, similarity to real-life drilling experience, and similarity to real-life microexploration. In addition, 96% of the participants stated that similar courses should be incorporated into official neurosurgical training programs.

Simulation courses offer a way to balance the growing need for comprehensive neurosurgical training with limited resources in LMICs. Through a distinctive blend of high-yield/low-risk investments, they possess the capability to transform neurosurgery education. In addition, utilizing digital simulation tools can offer a temporary solution to bridge the gap in neurosurgical training between developed countries and LMICs. These systems have advantages such as easy access, wide applicability, cost-effectiveness, and minimal need for human resources. Prior to integrating these courses into established neurosurgical curricula and expanding their use, it is necessary to conduct well-designed prospective studies that demonstrate a direct impact on patient safety and outcome measures.

Simulated Neurosurgery Using Animal Specimens in the Hoz Mentorship

So far, a total of 16 cranial neurosurgery techniques have been simulated on animal models that are not alive. Thus far, sheep, cows, and swine have been the three species of animals that are used. Animal training models exhibit anatomical variances in size, topographic anatomy, and neuronal structure when compared to humans and connections between blood vessels. Nevertheless, the models have a practical use by aiding trainees in developing their manual dexterity and to execute the surgical procedures associated with various cranial approaches. Furthermore, several of these distinctions are insignificant when considering microscopic surgery [7].

The course was implemented in the Hoz mentorship at the Neurosurgery Teaching Hospital in Baghdad. It aimed to expose medical students to high-yield neurosurgical procedures focusing on the indication of the procedure, anatomical considerations, technical steps and a comprehensive discussion about possible complications. The duration of this course was 7 hours that included two breaks in between. A total of thirty medical students were enrolled in this course. The facilitators are represented by the mentor, five senior neurosurgical residents and two graduated mentees. The course included four stations about significant neurosurgical procedures, these stations are:

- Station 1: Sheep cadaver station that was directed by two residents who explained the concept of craniotomy and burr hole-creating procedure. It also included a comprehensive overview of dura suturing techniques. The facilitators guided the mentees with steps to perform the procedure and evaluated their practical skills, scientific knowledge, and ethical behavior when working in teams.
- Station 2: Egg station, which included training the mentees about using microsurgical drills. This station aimed to enhance precision and aim-oriented hand skills. The facilitators of this station were a senior resident, and one graduated mentee who has meticulous talent in using the microsurgical drill.
- Station 3: Neurosurgical instruments station where the students are taught about the common instruments' names and indications in addition to differences and similarities between them. The resident who was responsible for this station provided the students with the opportunity to manually handle these instruments and try them on station 1.
- Station 4: Microsuturing station that involved the use of different suture materials like Nylon and silk with sizes ranging from 6-0 to 11-0. The station also included microsurgical loupes and offered the student simulation of the surgeon's perspective in dealing with microscopic neurosurgical procedures. The station was under the supervision of one resident and one graduated mentee.

The mentor was the Maestro who arranged all the elements of this course elegantly. He supervised the progress of every station and its level of clarity to the mentees. This book is not only about providing a structured mentorship model, it is also about explaining why you should never be alone in this journey of learning. Thus, the feelings of the mentees within this course are valuable and must be addressed properly. The hall of this course was big in a way that a person can stand at the end of it and sense the glory of its impact. A glory of the people who came to learn, who came to teach and who came to share. Despite the complexity of this course, the students were delighted and full of enthusiasm. Passion was contagious in that room. Different kind of gaze can be observed on their young faces. Curiosity gaze, analytical gaze, excitement gaze and astounded gaze. They were not only thrilled with the opportunity to learn but also were eager to support each other in understanding complex details. Each one of them has a different background and story. Maybe some of them had to walk alone in their lives, but not on that day. They witness a strange world where people can walk together hand in hand to serve humanity. Their intelligence is important, but sharing it can impact the public interest. They witness the true purpose of being a doctor and enjoy enriching their mind and skills to eventually deliver optimal patient care. The students were deeply grateful to the Maestro and his team for this uniquely influential day. It was brought to the attention of the students that there is a person who is enthusiastic about teaching neurosurgery and is willing to adapt his teaching style to various levels of intelligence among the mentees. Someone who is capable of organizing each and every detail with meticulousness. His moral visions and his boundless enthusiasm are captivating. His respect for more experienced surgeons is quite astounding. He imparted to the students the values of aspiration, compassion, and modesty. They were also grateful for the animals that were used to introduce them to the world of neurosurgery and optimize their hand skills. They will remember these animals every time they perform a successful burr hole to save their patients.

At the end of the day, the mentor and the director of the hospital presented each student with a certificate of participation showing that they had successfully completed this course. The collection of verbal feedback takes place in an environment that is very encouraging.

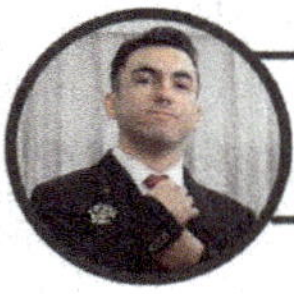

Mustafa Ismail

From my experience, Dr. Hoz's mentorship distills into two main principles: care and transformation. I engaged with Dr. Hoz mentorship for more than three years. First, I started with a naive perspective about clinical research and knowledge in neurosurgery. I was in medical school when I knew Dr. Hoz; then, all changed after we started interacting. Dr. Hoz insisted on pushing boundaries in research and neurosurgical knowledge. In the former, we opt to dig deeper into the spectacular topic of neurosurgery, which culminated in publishing more than 100 papers in peer-reviewed journals. For the latter, Dr. Hoz's perspective on neurosurgical knowledge is intricate and has multifaceted angles. The approach is pragmatic and based on real-world problems. He usually picks someone to attend in the operating room or the angiosuite, and then that person will develop a concrete understanding of the clinical case. This understanding is now an asset for investment and development. Dr. Hoz will assign him research subject to investigate and write about. This consolidation will deepen the understanding and nominate him to the next level.

The next phase is all about more care and transformation. When that someone was me, I had to manage 30 research projects simultaneously in my comfort zone. All I needed was to show interest and vacate my schedule. This process continued. After a while, I find myself in a completely different level. Different in the way I see and communicate. This transformation with care opened the doors for me. Currently, I am a researcher in the US with achievements that include 170 publications, four books, an editor and a reviewer in multiple high-impact journals. Dr. Hoz's touch has all that magic, so I deeply appreciate and thank my mentor.

Research course

All treatments, interventions, medications, methods of care, and post-treatment support in the healthcare system are derived from scientific discoveries. The exceptional level of care we have today is the result of extensive research and dedication by medical experts who have studied the various risk factors, causes, preventive measures, and therapies for diseases over many years. David Sackett, a prominent figure in the research field, provided a concise definition of evidence-based medicine (EBM) as "the conscientious, explicit, and judicious use of current best evidence in making decisions about the care of individual patients" [8]. EBM relies on scientifically produced information, which is methodically collected. This distinguishes it from subjective experience, which can be impacted by bias. Even the most qualified doctors might be influenced in their decision-making by recent patient experiences. Nevertheless, bias can be surmounted if the physician is receptive to the findings of extensive, well-regulated, and unbiased clinical trials that serve as the foundation for treatment approaches. The primary advantage of EBM is that it allows for the direct application of knowledge obtained from extensive clinical studies to patient care. The utilization of EBM ensures uniformity in the treatment of individual patients, with the expectation of achieving the best clinical results and enhancing their quality of life. One primary advantage of EBM is its application in the creation of evidence-based treatment guidelines. When analyzing prescribing patterns, it is advantageous to efficiently examine treatment strategies with physicians, emphasize the importance of the guidelines for managed care organizations (MCOs), and advocate for cost-effective formulary selections. By implementing data-Based Medicine (EBM) to reinforce clinical policy inside an organization, it becomes significantly more feasible to attain consensus among physicians regarding documented clinical data [9]. In order to achieve improved outcomes for patients with complex diseases, it is essential to focus on the development of treatment strategies that are based on evidence, as well as the education and training of physicians who are skilled in evaluating scientific literature perspective. Additionally, it is important for physicians to accept and adhere to EBM policies in a collaborative manner. The EBM concept is positioned to have a favorable influence in the managed care setting by delivering excellent medical care at a reduced cost and attaining optimal results.

The main aim of the Hoz research mentoring program is to enhance the management of neurosurgical illnesses on a global scale by doing high-quality research, providing exceptional clinical care, and offering comprehensive education. The team of medical researchers is committed to studying the etiology of diseases, developing improved therapeutic interventions, and effectively implementing the findings into novel clinical protocols. The approach is comprehensive, encompassing fundamental scientific study on the mechanisms of different neurosurgical disorders. The role entails conducting clinical investigations on novel medicines and creative methods for patient care, as well as implementing studies to enhance the adoption of our findings. The mentorship research initiatives also analyze extensive patient populations to ascertain the most effective public health methods for neurological well-being in our community. Our commitment to patients' wellness is vital to our mission.

This course is designed for medical students and neurosurgery residents who have a desire to make contributions in the field of research. The course aspect comprised the following:

- Medical research 101 demonstrates a fundamental understanding of the significance, classifications, and principles of medical research.

- Comprehensive elucidation of several study designs, such as descriptive and analytical. Furthermore, it included a comprehensive analysis of the objectives and practical uses of each method, as well as guidance on the process of selecting and designing a study. It also provided guidance on how to construct hypotheses.
- Instruction on how to read research papers, covering the significance of each section and the distinctions between them, including the abstract, introduction, method, result, discussion, and conclusion respectively
- Writing a research paper. The training initially focused on writing case reports. It then progressed to include writing review papers and subsequently expanded to encompass writing clinical study papers.
- Techniques for collecting data, approaches for assessing the reliability of each source, strategies for handling data collections, and methods for ensuring the accuracy of the data.
- Understanding the fundamentals of statistical analysis of data sets, as well as the various statistical software programs and how to interpret the results.
- Addressing the need to adhere to medical research ethics when working on research projects, such as obtaining informed consent, following research ethical guidelines, and receiving approval from Institutional Review Boards (IRB).

The class consists of three online lectures, with one lecture scheduled for each day of the week. Every lecture had a specific duration, after which the facilitator and mentees would participate in a discussion. After the session, each student was assigned a simple task to enhance their level of involvement. An additional component of the workshops was the invitation of a guest who discussed his or her experiences in gaining knowledge of medical research concepts and working on different research projects. Every student who successfully completed this course was allocated to a neurosurgical research project under the supervision of the mentor and facilitators. A significant number of these initiatives have been published in prestigious academic publications. At the very beginning of the mentorship, the mentor asked the students to search their names on searching database and save the result. Indeed, the results were devoid of any information. He promised them that their names would be known, and that the results section would be astounding. He is a man of his words and all of his statements are based on fact rather than a promise. Now, after a few years have passed, each one of them has compiled a list of publications that have inspired them and made them more determined to contribute to the field of medical research with the purpose of making better future for patients.

Resources for the Courses

The materials of each course differed according to multiple variables including the target audience and their goals. However, few resources were generally useful in each cycle of the Hoz Neurosurgery mentorship. Most of them were used to highlight anatomical or radiological points, in addition to neurosurgery related textbooks.

- Hoz Neurosurgery Youtube Channel
- The Neurosurgical Atlas by Aaron Cohen-Gadol, M.D. Youtube channel
- Snell's Clinical Neuroanatomy Textbook [10].
- Rhoton's Cranial Anatomy and Surgical Approaches Textbook [11].
- Greenberg's Handbook of Neurosurgery [12].
- Osborn's Brain [13].
- Prof. Mamdouh Mahfouz - Radiology
- Radiopedia

References

1. Konakondla S, Fong R, Schirmer CM. Simulation training in neurosurgery: advances in education and practice. Adv Med Educ Pract. 2017;8:465–73
2. Oliveira LM, Figueiredo EG. Simulation training methods in neurological surgery. Asian J Neurosurg. 2019;14(2):364–70.
3. Menna G, Kolias A, Esene IN, Barthélemy EJ, Hoz S, Laeke T, Silva AC, Longo-Calderón GM, Baticulon RE, Zabala JP, Hassani FD. Reducing the gap in neurosurgical education in LMICs: a report of a non-profit educational program. World Neurosurgery. 2024 Feb 1;182:e792-7.
4. Limbrick Jr DD, Dacey Jr RG. Simulation in neurosurgery: possibilities and practicalities: foreword. Neurosurgery. 2013 Oct 1;73:S1-3.
5. Bernardo A. Virtual reality and simulation in neurosurgical training. World Neurosurg. 2017;106:1015-1029.
6. Gasco J, Holbrook TJ, Patel A, et al. Neurosurgery simulation in residency training: feasibility, cost, and educational benefit. Neurosurgery. 2013;73(suppl 1):39-45.
7. Al-Sharshahi ZF, Hoz SS, Alrawi MA, Sabah MA, Albanaa SA, Moscote-Salazar LR. The use of non-living animals as simulation models for cranial neurosurgical procedures: a literature review. Chinese Neurosurgical Journal. 2020 Dec 10;6(04):230-4.
8. Lewis SJ, Orland BI. The importance and impact of Evidence Based Medicine. Journal of Managed Care Pharmacy. 2004 Sep;10(5 Supp A):S3-5.
9. Rodby RA, Orland BI, Lewis SJ, Hunsicker LG. An evidence-based approach: the emerging role of renal protection in hypertension; a focus on clinical and economic factors that impact formulary decision making. Journal of Managed Care Pharmacy. 2004 Sep;10(5 Supp A):1-32.
10. Snell RS. Clinical neuroanatomy. Lippincott Williams & Wilkins; 2010.
11. Rhoton Jr AL. Rhoton's cranial anatomy and surgical approaches. Oxford University Press; 2019 Oct 3.
12. Greenberg MS. Greenberg's handbook of neurosurgery. (No Title). 2023 Apr 19.

13. Osborn AG, Hedlund GL, Salzman KL. Osborn's brain e-book. Elsevier Health Sciences; 2017 Nov 2.

Section 1: Foundations of the Mentorship Program

CH.5: Implementing Hands-On Training and Clinical Rotations for Mentees

Rania H. Al-Taie, Aktham Osama Al-Khafaji, Teeba A. Al-Ageely

Section 1: Foundations of the Mentorship Program

CH.5: Implementing Hands-On Training and Clinical Rotations for Mentees

Early clinical exposure (ECE) is a strategy that combines the understanding of fundamental and clinical sciences with the psychological and social components of medical practice. Its purpose is to align medical education with the actual practice of medicine, resulting in the optimal training of competent physicians [1]. The significance of ECE is growing steadily on a daily basis. A study conducted by Başak et al. (2009) [2] revealed that ECE programs are being implemented in 40 medical schools across 16 European countries.

In accordance with the Graduate Medical Education Regulation of 2019, ECE was introduced as a novel element within the framework of Competency-Based Medical Education (CBME). Beginning with the 2019 cohort, this initiative was incorporated into the Medical curriculum. The primary objectives of implementing Early Clinical Exposure for first-year medical students are to enhance their capacity to recognize the importance of fundamental sciences in the areas of diagnosis, patient care, and treatment. Further, it provides a contextual framework that enhances students' understanding of fundamental scientific principles by directly connecting them to the experiential narratives of patients. ECE sessions provide medical students with a diverse range of motivations, enhancing their academic resilience, refining their clinical and communication abilities, and instilling self-assurance. From a scientific perspective, ECE represents a prime example of vertical integration, connecting the realms of preclinical and clinical subjects. This integration pattern not only strengthens theoretical knowledge through practical application but also fosters a comprehensive comprehension of medical concepts by integrating academic learning with real-world clinical experiences [3].

AkbariRad et al. (2023) [4] performed an empirical study on undergraduate medical students at Mashhad University of Medical Sciences, Mashhad, Iran, who were transitioning from the pre-clinical course to the externship course. The participants underwent an eight-session ECE intervention conducted by two professors from the Internal Medicine department. The participant's perception of the program and the program's quality were evaluated using a valid and reliable measure created by Mirzazadeh et al. (Cronbach's alpha = 0.72). The study included a cohort of

118 undergraduate medical students. The findings indicated that this program was successful in acquiring 81.2% of the students with the significance of fundamental scientific knowledge in clinical environments. Furthermore, 88.9% of the participants expressed their belief that this intervention had the potential to inspire them to pursue further studies. The statistics indicated that this curriculum was exceedingly captivating for international students. Based on the student's feedback, the program's main merits were providing exposure to clinical fields, offering exceptional professors, and delivering commendable instruction. Conversely, the program's primary drawback was its brief duration and the large number of participants in each group.

The Hoz Mentorship Early Clinical Exposure Model

Following the provision of essential theoretical knowledge to the mentees in online sessions and the subsequent selection of qualified students for clinical sessions based on straightforward competitive assessments, a number of students are chosen for the clinical experience. This course consists of four main stations, which include operating rooms, emergency rooms, intensive care units, and lab visits. Participants are usually divided into small groups to attend each section to prevent overcrowding and ensure optimal focus.

As an example of the application of this system, during the mentorship ninth cycle, a total of 10 students were chosen, and their clinical experience can be illustrated by phases (**Table 1**).

Phase 1 commenced with a total of 4 days, at a frequency of 2 days per week, taking place at the Neurosurgical Teaching Hospital in Baghdad, Iraq. The duration of each session is 12 hours. Indeed, all the students were enrolled in the clinical sessions. However, to ensure the safety of both the students and the patients, the remaining 10s students were enrolled after a period of 2 weeks, and this process continued thereafter. Since this initiative was taken during the pandemic in 2020, the students were required to present their immunization certificates and safety equipment, such as face masks and hand sanitizers. Additionally, they were instructed to bring their lab coats and notebooks. The medical staff supplied them with additional equipment, such as surgical gowns, gloves, surgical head covers, and shoe covers.

During the initial three days, four students are given access to the operating room, where they have the opportunity to see sophisticated neurosurgical operations, such as vascular neurosurgery, spine neurosurgery, and oncological neurosurgery. The students arrive promptly and begin by obtaining a concise medical history from the patient. They then carefully watch the necessary pre-operative preparations before donning sterilized scrubs. Once properly attired, they join the neurosurgical residents in the operating room to observe the procedure. A single neurosurgeon is responsible for providing an extensive overview of the surgical procedures to the students, ensuring that they get familiar with the process and the case operated on. Simultaneously, the students are encouraged to record their questions in their notebooks, which they can later share during the post-surgery discussion. Subsequently, they observe follow-up assessments of the patients to monitor their current status, and the mentor updates the students on a private online platform with the patient's daily progress. This approach aims to enhance the student's involvement with the patient's condition.

In the meantime, four students are assigned to the emergency room, where they acquire knowledge about fundamental concepts regarding obtaining medical history from patients, as well as basic principles of conducting physical examinations and reviewing systems. Additionally, they get knowledge on the basic concepts of hospital protocols, patient legal documentation, effective communication with patients and their companions, as well as recommendations for expressing empathy. Furthermore, this course covers fundamental concepts of clinical reasoning and provides an overview of the duties and responsibilities of staff members in hospitals and medical institutes. The last two students are assigned to the intensive care unit (ICU). The students acquired knowledge regarding the basic principles of critical care management, which encompass enhancing a patient's physiological state, delivering advanced organ support, and early diagnosing and treating underlying pathological conditions. They also learned about the role of a multidisciplinary team approach that involves shared responsibility between the admitting team and a specialist critical care team, which is supervised by a critical care physician. The students received focused instruction on the concepts and monitoring of intracranial pressure, the role of electroencephalogram (EEG), and advanced neurological monitoring in critically ill patients. The training also involved instruction on the concepts and techniques needed for administering the Glasgow Coma Scale (GCS) to assess the neurological condition of patients.

The process is similar each day, for which all ten students have the opportunity to visit the emergency room, ICU, and operating room. On the fourth day of the class, all students are assigned to different operating rooms and participate in the postoperative discussion. Then, the mentor receives their impressions and feedback.

The second phase of Early Clinical Exposure is introducing students to the radiological intervention department in the field of neurosurgery. This period spanned around three months, with two days per week. Each day, four students who have successfully completed phase 1 are chosen to observe endovascular neurosurgery. They had the opportunity to witness diagnostic techniques and minimally invasive therapeutic interventions for the treatment of various neurosurgical disorders, such as intracranial aneurysms and arteriovenous malformations. The trainees were educated on the advantages of endovascular neurosurgery, which include a shorter recovery period, reduced patient discomfort, smaller surgical incisions, less cardiovascular stress, and decreased risks for patients with various comorbidities. In addition, they were given details regarding the instruments and safety protocols.

Phase 3 consisted of a period of seven months spent in the operation room. Students who completed both Phase 1 and Phase 2 were given the opportunity to observe neurosurgical procedures at the Neurosurgery Teaching Hospital. This opportunity was available to four students per day, for two days each week, based on their availability and interest in pursuing a career in neurosurgery. Meanwhile, each individual is assigned to work on a research project that is relevant to the surgery they attended. Therefore, expanding their understanding through a diverse range of approaches.

Phase 4 was more of an advantageous phase where students take up vital clinical skills that could help with their careers in the future. Students were of tremendous aid in the emergency room; some students did some voluntary work in the emergency department in the neurosurgery teaching hospital in conditions where the resources were depleted, which was something doctors could regularly face in an LMIC, Iraq an example. This experience reflects the positive impact of mentees' training on their clinical skills and their capability to handle responsibility under pressure, which are vital characteristics for a future doctor.

Barriers to Clinical Training in the Hoz Neurosurgery Mentorship

Efficiency and adaptability are key goals of the mentorship program, and making informed decisions that contribute to overall success is essential. To attain success, it is crucial to prioritize the satisfaction of mentees, as it greatly impacts overall work accomplishments. This may be accomplished by maintaining a content and enthusiastic team as the driving force behind these endeavors. The cornerstone of a mentorship's value lies in its mentees. Nevertheless, cultivating professional advancement and progress is a continuous process that necessitates deliberate and thoughtful strategizing. This statement is particularly true when dealing with diverse challenges in student training and development.

There are many challenges and obstacles faced during the implication of this mentorship; an example is managing the impacts of change. Being the first medical mentorship program in Iraq has significant challenges. This major shift is accompanied by a variety of problems. The influence begins with the fundamental establishment of the mentorship, which involves obtaining approvals from the hospital director and the heads of the departments. Furthermore, an important concern is the students can occupy space in the operating rooms, emergency department, and ICU. This issue might have a detrimental impact on education and hinder the opportunity for neurosurgical residents to acquire knowledge and skills. Furthermore, it is important to consider the influence this has on students themselves, particularly their lack of knowledge regarding appropriate behavior in clinical practice. The approach we took to address this issue involves formulating a proposal that includes a comprehensive plan for the mentorship program, which then was presented to the relevant stakeholders. In addition, we restricted the number of students to an optimal capacity that allows for clinical training without compromising the training of residents. Furthermore, we involved the residents in the training of mentees by assigning them non-compulsory teaching tasks. And finally, during the online sessions, we conducted a presentation on "surgical etiquette" to instruct the students on appropriate behavior in clinical practice.

Another challenge is the financial barriers. Training can be an enormous commitment, particularly if you possess multiple units and need to train students at various locations. The expenses can rapidly accumulate, encompassing the cost of both materials and trainers. Indeed, the quality of the training program should not be compromised by its cost. Adopting a well-balanced approach can lead to outstanding outcomes without incurring excessive costs. Effective and economical training can be achieved through strategic planning and resource allocation. We addressed this issue by leveraging online platforms in order to minimize expenses associated with physical training materials and venues. In addition, our team of skilled professionals provides voluntary training to the students. Furthermore, we have established partnerships with organizations such as UpSurgeon, which have reduced the training materials expenses. We also have adopted a group training technique to optimize the utilization of the time and resources.

Furthermore, time restriction is another issue encountered during these courses. Efficient time management is essential for executing a solid training program without disrupting the studying process. Strategically scheduling and organizing training sessions can effectively uphold productivity while ensuring that students acquire essential skills. By dividing the training into smaller, more manageable modules that can be completed during downtime, we were able to resolve this issue.

In order to provide a more flexible scheduling plan, we integrated online and in-person training. In an attempt to mitigate disruptions, we also conducted the training sessions on days off. Ultimately, we implemented software that utilized time-tracking tools to closely monitor the time spent on training activities.

Another example of the commonly faced challenges is the retention of skill. The purpose of training is not only to impart skills but rather to ensure that these skills are kept and properly utilized in clinical practice. Retaining skills can provide a considerable problem, particularly when students are inundated with a large amount of information rapidly. To ensure that students retain what they have learned, we have considered implementing ways to enhance memory retention and skill application. Consequently, we have developed a communication system that allows students to request assistance or clarification even after the completion of the training time. In addition, we provided regular and comprehensive reviews to strengthen previously acquired skills. Furthermore, we offered students the chance to put into practice the knowledge they have acquired in a supervised setting.

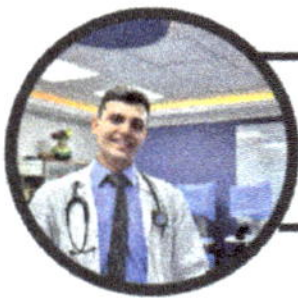

Mahmood F. Al-Zaidy

"I believe that a surgeon who discovers a passion for a specialty early is more likely to excel and develop bey their peers."

This was the statement I wrote in my cover letter when applying for the mentorship program, shortly a completing the first stage of medical school. At the time, I knew only one thing with certainty I had dreamed becoming a neurosurgeon since childhood. However, I was unsure of how or where to begin. Being accepted a mentee, and as the youngest among those selected, marked the start of a transformative journey. Determined make the most of this opportunity, I committed myself to simultaneously learn the fundamentals of medicine a neurosurgery, striving to demonstrate persistence, dedication, and genuine passion for the field.

A pivotal moment came when I was selected for what we called "SWAT 1 team", where I was one of six ment granted access to the emergency room, intensive care unit, and neurosurgical operating rooms. This marked true beginning of my clinical experience. Under the guidance of Dr. Hoz, my mentor, I gained invaluable expos to operating room protocols, radiographic interpretation, surgical procedures, and hands-on training in the surgi skills lab. This period was not only rich in knowledge but also filled with unforgettable experiences that deepe my passion for neurosurgery. I found myself particularly drawn to the clinical and surgical aspects of the specia attending and actively participating in operations, following up on patients, and engaging in direct patient car an aspect I cherished the most.

From the beginning of my mentorship until now, I have attended and participated in over 150 craniotomy and sp surgeries, along with more than 75 diagnostic and therapeutic cerebral endovascular procedures. Throughout journey, I have gained profound insights into neurosurgical conditions, surgical techniques, and pati management. However, one of the most valuable skills I developed was the ability to perform under pressure as essential trait in this demanding specialty.

Beyond clinical training, one of the most significant aspects of my mentorship was research. Under Dr. Ho guidance, I engaged in numerous research projects across various domains, often taking on leadership roles. mentorship in scientific writing and research methodology provided me with a strong foundation, shaping academic career. Today, I have contributed to over 20 publications, including books and research papers achievement made possible through his support and dedication.

Joining the mentorship program and working under Dr. Hoz's leadership was the most defining experience of clinical and academic journey. His guidance not only accelerated my growth but also set me on the right p saving me years of uncertainty. He was more than a mentor he was a guiding force who shaped my aspirations a helped me navigate the complexities of neurosurgery with confidence and purpose.

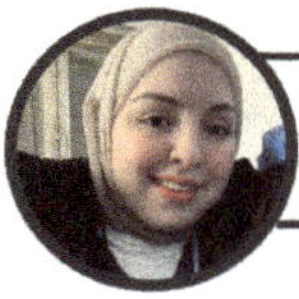

Fatimah O. Al-Hashimi

ne moments in life shape us in ways we never expect. Looking back, I realize that my journey into neurosurgery s built on a series of defining experiences, each one pushing me further and sharpening my vision of the doctor I nted to become.

: first time I met Dr. Hoz was during my second year of medical college, and it completely changed my perspective what it means to be a doctor. In this program, we were taught the science and hand skills necessary for neurosurgery also offered the invaluable opportunity to engage with international neurosurgeons, where we were encouraged to k beyond traditional practices trying to bridge the gaps between the local and international standards.

at struck me the most was his vision. He often spoke of **"Kaizen"**, a Japanese term meaning "continuous provement," and it resonated deeply with me. Dr. Hoz's relentless determination to improve the reality of medicine s evident in everything he did. He didn't settle for practicing within the confines of a low-to-middle-income country. : Baghdad Neurovascular Center (BNC) was proof of that. I always feel privileged that I have witnessed the ndation of one of Iraq's first neurovascular centers, a place dedicated to pushing boundaries, integrating ernational expertise, and creating invaluable opportunities for students and residents to grow.

my fifth year, after my very first visit to the BNC, I knew that I wanted to attend more sessions and become a part this team. The work-study load was intense, but it was exactly what I was searching for. Hoz and his residents started by teaching me the basics—learning anatomy, understanding procedures, niliarizing myself with the equipment. But within days, I was passing on that knowledge to other students, guiding m through discussions on anatomy, procedural steps, and technical set-ups.

: Baghdad-KSA meetings provided a comprehensive learning experience, combining intraoperative guidance with depth pre- and post-operative online meetings. The live intraoperative proctoring refined our technical abilities and blem-solving approach, teaching us how to anticipate, address, and overcome complications in real time. Beyond technical aspects, the pre- and post-operative discussions offered a deeper understanding of surgical decision-king. These meetings went beyond procedural steps, focusing on anticipating challenges, planning for potential nplications, strategizing solutions, and selecting the best treatment options—not just from a medical standpoint, but) considering financial factors. Engaging in these discussions has exposed me to an advanced decision-making cess that most students never get to experience. Ultimately, they shaped my understanding of what it truly means to a neurosurgeon—not just someone who performs surgeries, but someone who thinks critically, adapts, and ovates.

naturing moment came when we were short-staffed during a procedure, and I had to step up and take on several nnical tasks. This experience taught me how to synchronize into the operating room's harmony, anticipate the next ps, and adapt to unexpected challenges, which ultimately boosted my confidence and solidified my role within the n. It was a moment of realization—I wasn't just gaining skills; I was developing the mindset required to operate in h-stakes environments.

w, as a junior resident in an academic medical center in Baghdad, I see the impact of those experiences every day. : discipline, confidence, and professionalism I developed at BNC set me apart among my peers. Senior doctors trust with their patients, knowing that I handle cases with precision and responsibility. My ability to navigate urgent ations, communicate effectively with senior physicians, and contribute meaningfully to team discussions has ome a defining aspect of my work.

ur duty in life is to support each other and make the next generation even better," Dr. Hoz often said, and lived hat philosophy every day. That message has stayed with me ever since. If there's one lesson I've truly internalized n this, it's: real success isn't about what you accomplish alone—it's about how many people you help rise with you.

Table 1: A Structured, Multi-Phase Approach to Early Clinical Exposure in Neurosurgery

Phase	Duration & Schedule	Key Focus Areas	Activities	Educational Outcomes
Phase 1: Foundational Clinical Exposure	4 days over 2 weeks (2 days per week, 12 hours per session)	Introduction to Clinical Settings (Operating Room, Emergency Room, ICU)	- Operating Room: Observing advanced neurosurgical procedures (vascular, spine, oncological surgeries). - Emergency Room: Understanding patient interaction (history taking, basic physical exams, legal documentation). - ICU: Learning critical care management (intracranial pressure, GCS, EEG monitoring).	- Familiarity with neurosurgical procedures and protocols. - Development of clinical reasoning and patient interaction skills. - Understanding the fundamentals of critical care and multidisciplinary team coordination.
Phase 2: Specialized Radiology Exposure	3 months (2 days per week, 4 students per session)	Advanced Diagnostic & Therapeutic Techniques in Neurosurgical Radiology	- Observing radiological interventions and minimally invasive procedures (e.g., endovascular treatment of aneurysms, arteriovenous malformations). - Understanding the role of endovascular neurosurgery and its advantages in patient care.	- In-depth knowledge of diagnostic imaging techniques. - Learning about minimally invasive therapeutic interventions and their benefits (reduced recovery time, smaller incisions, etc.). - Mastery of radiological safety protocols.
Phase 3: Intensive Surgical and Research Integration	7 months (2 days per week, 4 students per session)	Focused Surgical Exposure & Research Application	- Extended observation of neurosurgical procedures at the Neurosurgical Teaching Hospital. - Simultaneous involvement in research projects aligned with observed surgeries, enhancing academic and clinical integration.	- Advanced understanding of neurosurgical techniques. - Application of clinical knowledge to research, developing critical thinking and investigative skills. - Cultivating a deeper interest in neurosurgical research and practice.
Phase 4: Practical Skills Development & Volunteering	Flexible, based on availability and ongoing throughout the mentorship	Practical Application & Leadership in Resource-Limited Settings	- Participation in emergency room activities under high-pressure conditions (e.g., resource shortages). - Hands-on involvement in patient care and team-based problem-solving in low-resource environments typical of LMICs like Iraq.	- Enhanced clinical decision-making and leadership skills under pressure. - Building resilience and adaptability in emergency care settings. - Real-world exposure to common challenges in healthcare systems in low- and middle-income countries.

References

1. Tayade MC, Latti RG. Effectiveness of early clinical exposure in medical education: Settings and scientific theories–Review. Journal of Education and Health Promotion. 2021 Jan 1;10(1):117.
2. Başak O, Yaphe J, Spiegel W, Wilm S, Carelli F, Metsemakers JF. Early clinical exposure in medical curricula across Europe: an overview. The European journal of general practice. 2009 Jan 1;15(1):4-10.
3. Verma M. Early clinical exposure: New paradigm in Medical and Dental Education. Contemporary clinical dentistry. 2016 Jul 1;7(3):287-8.
4. AkbariRad M, Khadem-Rezaiyan M, Ravanshad S, Rafiee M, Firoozi A, Zolfaghari SA, Aghaei HR, Zadehahmad R, Azarkar S, Moodi Ghalibaf A. Early clinical exposure as a highly interesting educational program for undergraduate medical students: an interventional study. BMC Medical Education. 2023 May 1;23(1):292.

Section 2: Collaborative and Research Initiatives

CH.6: Strengthening the Hoz Mentorship Program through Global SNI Collaborations

Rania H. Al-Taie, Ali M. Neamah, Teeba A. Al-Ageely, Mohammed A. Al-Dhahir, Samer S. Hoz

Section 2: Collaborative and Research Initiatives

CH.6: Strengthening the Hoz Mentorship Program through Global SNI Collaborations

Surgical Neurology International (SNI) has been actively involved in providing knowledge about disorders of the central nervous system that are relevant to all scientists since 2010. Neurosurgeons, neurologists, epidemiologists, and researchers from all countries study the papers published in the SNI. Based on their extensive personal experience interacting with individuals from other countries, including those with lower and intermediate incomes, they have observed the presence of brilliant and innovative individuals worldwide. In 2021, the platform of SNI™ expanded and a 2-day educational summit on neurosurgical sub-specialties was hosted under a new educational system funded by SNI Digital. The speakers are from many countries around the world. The participation of neurosurgeons from low- and middle-income countries (LMIC) was remarkable. Neurosurgeons from high-income nations communicated with colleagues from low- and middle-income countries regardless of any assumed differences in technology. Experts from several countries discussed the management of trauma, spine disease, epilepsy, pediatric neuro-oncology, vascular disease, and functional disease. They established other conduits of information that were not previously utilized, such as journals and static meetings. The prioritization of information discourse proved to be more significant than the mere accumulation of additional information, as it facilitated the development of more comprehensive viewpoints on each respective topic matter. SNI Digital™ has supported the global education of neurosurgeons, including both young neurosurgeons and students, in over 100 trial programs. These activities consist of interactive lectures, research evaluations, student presentations, grand rounds, and case discussions, led by both local and international instructors, catering to individuals of all age groups. Collaborative research endeavors involving people from several countries have resulted in the publication of scholarly papers. All sessions have been done via the Zoom platform, facilitating discussions among the participants. This initiative is an emerging global communication program that can be developed or modified based on the input of volunteers and the requirements of the observers [1].

SNI/SNI Digital-Baghdad neurosurgery educational series

The establishment of educational programs in a nation following years of internal conflicts, division, and external war is a formidable task. The high significance of neurosurgery in Iraq is attributed to the high incidence of head injuries that occur during wartime. SNI Digital/Surgical Neurology International (SNI) is collaborating to organize educational experiences. The audience's participation in these presentations is essential for achieving a satisfying educational experience. One of the most prevalent learning instruments on a global scale is the use of online educational methods [2,3]. Nevertheless, Iraq is included in the category of low- and middle-income countries that have limited access to high-quality neurosurgery online learning. The necessity for global collaboration and connection to facilitate the exchange of ideas and experiences among neurosurgeons is a challenge, but it is highly advantageous in that it broadens the scope of various perspectives on any subject. The meetings consisted of the following activities:

- Lectures that presented clinical experiences of neurosurgeons from worldwide and discussions regarding challenges and future directions.
- The presentation of research work and discussion of the fundamentals of forming research questions, in addition to the design of methods for solving those questions.
- Discussions and sharing of knowledge in various areas such as social, political, cultural, and management aspects relating to people. This was done to enhance the educational experience and tailor it to the specific needs of the local community.

A total of twelve monthly meetings took place from May 2021 to April 2022, with each session lasting up to 2 hours. The subsequent sessions were documented for individuals who were unable to participate in the regular gatherings. In fact, the attendees of the SNI-Baghdad meeting included a wide range of individuals, including medical students and attending neurosurgeons. The ratio of males to females was equal, with a 1:1 proportion. Approximately 90% of the participants found Professor Lazareff's presentations on research concepts to be beneficial, while 80% gave excellent ratings to the post-presentation conversations. Approximately 50-65% of individuals reported an enhancement in their ability to generate research ideas, evaluate existing material, and compose academic articles as a result of these interactions. One of the main goals of the SNI-Baghdad project is to enhance the ability of medical students to confidently deliver presentations on a case or research topic in a public setting. 85.8% of participants indicated that these sessions have influenced their career planning and enhanced their professional development by providing opportunities for strategic thinking. These discussions provide medical students with an encouraging message that they may successfully accomplish their goals with effective preparation and skills, and can enhance their ability to achieve these goals in the future [4]. Inclusive discussions based on factual information aimed at reaching logical conclusions have the greatest likelihood of success in any society. Furthermore, the Golden Rule, "Do unto others as you would want done unto you," is a fundamental principle that underpins the success of all communities. In order to ensure a promising future, it is imperative to capitalize on the finest aspects of our cultural legacy and foster mutual growth and collaboration.

SNI Impacts on Iraqi Medical Students

The collaboration of pioneers in the field of neurosurgery to enhance the knowledge of medical practitioners worldwide is a profoundly inspiring phenomenon on many levels. This may be attributed not only to the development of scientific knowledge but also to the active involvement of these innovators who generously impart their experience and dedicate their time to guiding students and residents, thereby fostering their growth and progress. These neurosurgeons are committed to spreading innovation to many parts of the world and they have faith in the potential of everyone, irrespective of their backgrounds.

The students experienced a sense of companionship, no longer feeling as if they were walking alone. This feeling would arise throughout the early days of the mentorship clinical training, and it would continue to grow on a global level. The situation seemed to involve influential individuals strolling together along a single path. This is the path of innovation. The destination of this road is grand and impressive. It represents the process of optimizing the quality of treatment provided to patients. The student used to experience a sense of being left behind as he observed other medical students in high-income countries thriving in a well-structured learning environment. Then in these meetings, he attentively obtained an encouraging review of his work from these neurosurgeons, which provided him with significant support. He is currently optimistic and enthusiastic about further growth. He now realizes the wisdom of his mentor's statement: "Doing more with less."

Indicating that we can achieve great results with very few resources. In addition, he is observing a man who is proactively searching out learning opportunities for himself, his residents, and his mentees. This individual is willing to go above and beyond for them without hesitation or special benefit. The motivation was contagious throughout these meetings. We were concerned on behalf of our colleague who was going to present his/her ideas and work to surgeons from around the world. We possessed sufficient confidence to engage in the discussion. This confidence is derived from the guidance and support we received through the mentorship, which equipped us with knowledge and moral lessons that strengthened us. Subsequently, when our colleague receives favorable evaluations and significant recommendations from esteemed scientists, we together celebrate and strengthen one another. These scientists highlighted the significance of acknowledging that each patient is unique and that we should always remember there is a person behind the pathology. Indeed, the following is a summary of lessons that we have acquired from them:

- The only person you are behind is walking an identical path to yours, and such a person does not exist.
- Innovation extends beyond identity, religion, race, and gender. Your intelligence is both valid and distinctive, and no force can repress it. Under proper guidance, you will acquire the knowledge and skills necessary to enhance and strengthen your chosen path.
- Sharing is an act of demonstrating care for others. Possessing extensive expertise is beneficial, but imparting this knowledge to someone in need is truly exceptional. Imagine having a bag filled with seeds and spotting an empty land with fertile soil. You choose to plant these seeds there, and eventually, you behold an attractive and glowing nature.
- You rise by raising the people around you. Our mentor demonstrated this by exerting a significant amount of effort to connect us with international scientists to inspire us and expand our knowledge.
- Research is not only a task we need to do as doctors. It is a responsibility that we were assigned to it by our communities. These meetings taught us to be researchers who not only seek answers but also seek the best ways of serving our patients.

Implementation of SNI Meetings in the Hoz Mentorship

The proportion of online learners participating in virtual meetings has increased significantly in the past decade, and it has grown even more significantly during the COVID-19 pandemic [5]. In theory, these meetings have the potential to enhance neurosurgery, training, and standards in low- and middle-income countries including Iraq by acquiring the experience of developed countries. The growing number of online meetings across various platforms presents unique obstacles. One of the challenges is the maintenance of periodic online meetings that are of a consistent quality and that engage participants. The online meeting approach of the Surgical Neurology International (SNI®, SNI Digital™)-Baghdad neurosurgery (SNI-B meeting) has maintained exceptional consistency in both the frequency and quality of virtual meetings for over a year, based on our experience. The panel of discussants for the SNI involved Drs. J. Ausman, J. Lazareff, S. A. Khonsary, and A. Bari. Each individual has participated in educational endeavors abroad, spanning over more than 80 countries. They possessed an understanding and perceptiveness regarding the cultural disparities among individuals in numerous nations.

Prior to the live meeting, three virtual meetings took place between the faculty of SNI and Dr. Hoz to strategize various components of the meeting. Dr. Hoz made comprehensive local plans to adhere to the country's customs and to invite prominent speakers. The meeting was conducted virtually using the Zoom platform. The meeting was recorded for accessibility on SNI®. SNI Digital™ post-meeting available for public viewing. The mp4 recording of the meeting was sent out to the mentees, Iraqi neurosurgeons, as well as to professionals in other medical disciplines, for their reference. The entirety of the discussions took place in the English language. A group of speakers were chosen to present their work, which was then followed by a dynamic and interactive conversation including both the panel and the attendees.

At the fifteenth meeting, neurosurgeons from all generations engaged in discussions regarding their own experiences. Dr. A. Hadi Al Khalili, a pioneer in the field of neurosurgery in Iraq, was the first speaker [6]. Throughout his career in Iraq, spanning from the 1970s to 2004, he conducted extensive scientific research and engaged in enormous clinical practice. Furthermore, Dr. Moneer K. Faraj, the current chair of the local committee of the Arabian Board of Neurosurgery-Iraq, gave a presentation. Next speaker was Dr. Hiba AbdulAmeer who established her position as the youngest Arabic neurosurgeon up till now. Currently, she is an actively practicing neurosurgeon in Iraq. Next, Dr. Ausaf A. Bari, a functional neurosurgeon-scientist from the University of California, Los Angeles (UCLA) in the United States, gave a lecture. The conclusion of the meeting was devoted to a round of inquiries and responses including the discussants, instructors, and students. The primary motivation for the majority of registrants is a strong interest in learning about neurosurgery. The study involved a total of 17 neurosurgeons, 15 residents, and 28 medical students who had a specific interest in neurosurgery. Various interactive inquiries, responses, and recommendations were shared among the participants and deliberated upon at the conclusion of the gathering. These questions are appealing because of the wide range of individuals they attract, including both experienced neurosurgeons and medical students in the early stages of their education. The various levels of exploration create a constellation of thought-provoking questions that have the potential to enhance the understanding of anyone who is attentive. The attendees' response to this meeting was exceptionally positive. The majority of attendees concluded that the 15th SNI-Baghdad neurosurgery online meeting had a transformative impact on their perspective of neurosurgery [7]. Although we faced challenges during the meeting, they were inconsequential to the audience. Common technical issues that people have grown accustomed to present obstacles as do certain aspects of modern technology that lack user-friendliness. The speakers exceeded the anticipated duration of their presentations. However, the responses were irrelevant, yet it is necessary to address the issue in the future.

Interactive education entails comprehending the needs of the audience and delivering the necessary information to fulfill those needs. It entails a compassionate regard for students of all ages. The educational environment should be enjoyable and pleasant in order to foster a lifelong appealing experience, so ensuring that reading, learning, and exploration remain consistently captivating. The objective underlying this concept is to always remember the experience of being a medical student since it fosters a sense of companionship among individuals in diverse roles. The entire foundation is rooted in the principle of prioritizing the optimal course of action for the patient.

Who are the SNI Meetings' Faculty?

The panel involved four main figures who have reputable experience in the neurosurgery and research fields. The leading professor was Dr. James I. Ausman, MD, PhD, is an internationally renowned neurosurgeon, educator, and visionary in both the medical and business worlds. Known for his pioneering work in cerebrovascular surgery and brain tumors.

A Phi Beta Kappa graduate from Tufts University, Dr. Ausman earned his MD from Johns Hopkins University School of Medicine, where he was among a selected group of students awarded their degree in three years instead of the traditional four. He furthered his education at SUNY Buffalo, earning an MS in Physiology while completing a Cancer Research Fellowship at Roswell Park Memorial Cancer Institute. Dr. Ausman's training as a neurosurgeon was completed at the University of Minnesota, where he was one of five recipients of the National Institutes of Health (NIH) Teacher-Investigator five-year scholarship awards. He also earned a PhD in Pharmacology from George Washington University.

Dr. Ausman's academic career is distinguished by his tenure as Professor of Neurosurgery at the University of Michigan, University of Illinois at Chicago, and the University of Minnesota. He led the Departments of Neurosurgery at Henry Ford Hospital in Detroit and the University of Illinois in Chicago.

Dr. Ausman has written over 600 books and scientific publications. He has been invited as a Visiting Professor and neurosurgeon to 70 countries, primarily in LMIC. He is also a pioneer in the development of surgical techniques and microsurgical instruments. He founded the first Brain Tumor Support group for patients and their families and has educated over 400 neurosurgeons from more than 90 countries, with many of his trainees assuming leadership roles in their respective nations.

Recognized internationally, Dr. Ausman has received numerous awards, including the French Society of Arts, Sciences, and Letters. Three international libraries have been named in his honor, further solidifying his legacy in the field of neurosurgery. Dr. Jorge A. Lazareff is a highly esteemed neurosurgeon based in Los Angeles, California, with over 45 years of experience in the medical field. He is widely recognized for his contributions to both neurosurgery and medical education.

In 2014, Dr. Lazareff initiated a pioneering program aimed at fostering clinical research by introducing medical students and graduates to the principles of Critical Thinking, particularly in the interpretation of clinical evidence. This innovative program has been implemented in several medical schools across Latin America, including Guatemala, Costa Rica, and El Salvador, and has since expanded to Peru and Nicaragua. The course, which consists of seven lectures delivered in Spanish via the Internet, has equipped numerous students with essential skills in clinical research.

Dr. Lazareff's impact on global medical education has been further acknowledged through several prestigious honors. In 2019, he was awarded an Honorary Degree in Medicine from the Universidad Nacional Autónoma de Nicaragua (UNAN-Managua). In 2022, he was appointed

Docente Extraordinario by the Universidad Científica del Sur in Lima, Peru, in recognition of his outstanding contributions to medical academia.

Throughout his career, Dr. Lazareff has published over 100 peer-reviewed articles and research papers, making significant contributions to the field of neurosurgery. His work, which has garnered widespread attention with numerous citations, continues to influence the development of medical research and education in Latin America.

Dr. Seyed Ali Khonsary is a distinguished expert in the field of neurosurgery, known for his extensive contributions to both clinical practice and academic research. With a career spanning several decades, Dr. Khonsary has gained a reputation for his expertise in complex neurosurgical procedures and his dedication to advancing medical knowledge. Dr. Khonsary has made significant contributions to the neurosurgical field through his research, with his publications and numerous citations to his credit. His work covers a broad range of topics, with a particular focus on advancing surgical techniques and improving patient outcomes. Dr. Khonsary's research has been highly regarded in the scientific community, where his contributions continue to shape current medical practices. Dr. Khonsary remains a leader in his field, continually advancing the boundaries of neurosurgical research and education.

Dr. Abdul Hadi Al-Khalili is a pioneering figure in neurosurgery in Iraq, whose impact on the field has been profound and far-reaching. Born in Al-Kufa, Iraq, on May 11, 1943, Dr. Al-Khalili was raised in a family steeped in medicine, science, and law. His early fascination with the doctor-patient relationship, cultivated in his father's clinic, guided him toward a career in medicine.

Dr. Al-Khalili obtained his medical degree from the University of Baghdad in 1966. Initially specializing in ophthalmology in the United Kingdom, he later switched to neurosurgery, training at prestigious institutions such as Pinderfields Hospital in Yorkshire and the General Infirmary in Leeds. He became a Fellow of the Royal College of Surgeons and earned a master's degree in the philosophy of science from the University of Bradford. Upon completing his neurosurgery training in 1976, Dr. Al-Khalili returned to Iraq, where he became a leader in neurosurgery, known for his academic leadership and international collaborations.

Throughout his career, Dr. Al-Khalili has contributed to the field of neurosurgery in various ways. He invented the "Baghdadi Cerebral Hydatid Cyst Evacuation Instrument" in 1987, a groundbreaking tool used in the treatment of cerebral hydatidosis, a disease that was once referred to as "The Cancer of Iraq." He also established the first advanced Orbital Surgery Center in

Baghdad in 2002, recognized by the World Health Organization and the American Academy of Ophthalmology. In addition to his clinical innovations, Dr. Al-Khalili has been a strong advocate for modernizing neurosurgical practices in Iraq, introducing international standards and computerized patient data systems. His efforts have shaped the neurosurgical landscape of the country, even as he practiced through three consecutive wars, demonstrating resilience and ingenuity. After 2004, Dr. Al-Khalili served as the Iraqi cultural attaché in the United States, continuing to support the development of healthcare in Iraq. His legacy, marked by his leadership, inventions, and dedication to patient care, remains a cornerstone in the history of neurosurgery in Iraq. [7,8].

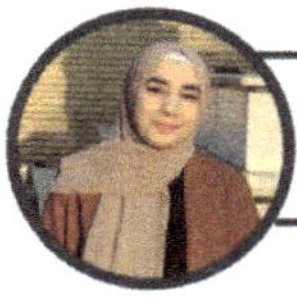

Noor M. Akar

As a first-generation medical student, my path was initially filled with uncertainty, navigating the complexitie medicine without guidance. However, the mentorship experience became a true turning point in my journey—it op countless doors and taught me invaluable lessons, not just academically but also in my personal and professional I learned how to manage my time effectively. I used to think productivity required long hours, but I discovered smart work is the key—knowing how to make the most of even short periods to achieve great results. I atte numerous surgeries, both catheter-based and open procedures, and was part of the team during some of the complex and challenging operations. Inside the operating room, I observed and learned from highly skilled, professi doctors, gaining exposure to intricate details in various surgical specialties.

These experiences inspired me to dive into research and writing. I published over seven works, including books articles in different fields. This was a huge step for me because it proved that I could contribute meaningfully t scientific community. I also delivered several presentations, one of the most important being at the SNI confere That opportunity was one of the greatest I've ever had—not just because I was able to present on a global platform because it allowed me to connect with leading doctors in neuroscience field and build meaningful professi relationships.

One memorable experience was when I wrote a presentation in just fifteen minutes and delivered it confidently. taught me how to stay calm and perform well under pressure, proving to myself that I could rise to any challeng matter how tough. Throughout this period, I learned the importance of teamwork and how to collaborate effective became calmer in my thinking, decision-making, and overall approach to work, which has reflected positively not in my studies but in my daily life as well.

This mentorship was the first structured guidance program I participated in. Despite hoz mentor's demanding sche as a neurosurgeon—and as the first Iraqi doctor specializing in cerebral vascular surgery—he always made tin guide us. We had daily meetings, whether group sessions or individual check-ins for students who needed advi direction. This consistent support was a powerful motivator for me to push my limits and continuously improve.

What made this experience even more special was that it wasn't limited to students from my country. I was part international community, engaging with students from various countries. I learned how they think, what they air and how their educational systems function. This broadened my perspective and helped me think more glob Through this mentorship, I had the opportunity to join the Dandy project, which became one of the most valu experiences I've had. Working on this project enriched my knowledge and skills, and I received st recommendations that continue to benefit me in my career. But the mentorship wasn't just about academics—it be a platform for me to explore my other passions. During this time, I learned digital illustration, and one of my draw was published in the Dandy project. That was a proud moment for me, as I managed to merge my passion for art my medical career. Additionally, I learned design skills and became the designer for more than five presentations d mentorship meetings. I was responsible for designing presentations for major conferences like SNI and Neurosu TV, which significantly boosted my confidence in my creative and organizational abilities.

My mentorship experience wasn't just an academic milestone—it was a journey of self-discovery and the beginni a career filled with passion and ambition. I learned how to stay focused, face challenges with confidence, and, importantly, believe in my abilities while striving to achieve my goals, no matter the obstacles.

References

1. Lazareff J, Hoz SS, Ausman JI, Al-Khalili AH, Khonsary SA, Epstein NE. Wanted: Volunteers to help people throughout the world. Surg Neurol Int 2023;14:63.
2. Correia AP, Liu C, Xu F. Evaluating videoconferencing systems for the quality of the educational experience. Distance Educ 2020;41:429-52. 3.
3. Hoz SS, Ismail M, Almufadhal MH, Al-Ageely TA, Aljuboori Z. Reinvigorating medical student mentorships in neurosurgery during the pandemic: Lessons learned from Iraq. Surg Neurol Int 2022;13.
4. Ismail M, Al-Ageely TA, Abdualmurtafie ZI, Daily SK, Ayad F, Al Khafaji AO, et al. SNI/SNI Digital-Baghdad neurosurgery educational series. Surg Neurol Int 2022;13:485.
5. Karl KA, Peluchette JV, Aghakhani N. Virtual work meetings during the COVID-19 pandemic: The good, bad, and ugly. Small group research. 2022 Jun;53(3):343-65.
6. Al-Sharshahi ZF, Al-Hemiery HA, Albaqer HA, Hamandi YM, Al-Awadi OM, Hoz SS. Following the footprints of pioneers on neurosurgery in Iraq: Abdul Hadi Al-Khalili. Surgical Neurology International. 2021;12.
7. Ismail M, Ahmed FO, Abdulsada AM, Al-Khafaji AO, Hoz SS, Lazareff JA, Khonsary SA, Ausman JI. "The most inspiring and mind-blowing meetings ever:" Highlights of the 15th SNI Baghdad Neurosurgery Online Meeting, from Participants' Perspectives. Surgical Neurology International. 2022;13.
8. Al-Sharshahi ZF, Al-Hemiery HA, Albaqer HA, Hamandi YM, Al-Awadi OM, Hoz SS. Following the footprints of pioneers on neurosurgery in Iraq: Abdul Hadi Al-Khalili. Surgical Neurology International. 2021;12.

Section 2: Collaborative and Research Initiatives

CH.7: Building Regional Partnerships through Baghdad–KSA Neurosurgery Projects

Rania H. Al-Taie, Sura H Talib, Haneen A. Salih, Teeba A. Al-Ageely, Samer S. Hoz

Section 2: Collaborative and Research Initiatives

CH.7: Building Regional Partnerships through Baghdad–KSA Neurosurgery Projects

Surgical proctoring, which involves the process of observing, supervising, and instructing experienced professionals, plays an important role in multiple fields [1]. Proctoring is a widely recognized tool in the field of neuroendovascular surgery. Nevertheless, the swift progress in equipment, along with imaging and surgical technologies, requires the presence of a conveniently available network of proctors [2,3]. The lack of in-person proctoring is particularly prominent in areas like Iraq, where multiple variables lead to a significantly limited availability of neuroendovascular training. These problems encompass a shortage of specialists in the domain, the exorbitant expenses of supplies and equipment for patients due to the absence of medical insurance in Iraq, and the inherent challenges linked to traveling to an area affected by war.

The KSA-Baghdad Program Setting

The Baghdad Neurovascular Center (BNC) is the first neurovascular institution in Iraq that combines different elements, and it was created in 2021. The BNC performs a diverse array of neurovascular treatments, including both open cerebrovascular surgery and diagnostic/therapeutic procedures. The surgical team at the center consists of five vascular neurosurgeons who have received training in both vascular surgery and neurosurgery. The leader of the team is the same leader of this mentorship, Dr. Samer S. Hoz who has a remarkable three-month endovascular fellowship experience in Japan, while the other team members have gained their competence by self-training within the team. Furthermore, the team involves numerous medical students and residents who contribute to the collaborative effort. Two operative rooms are completely equipped within the BNC. Specifically, one room is designated for open vascular neurosurgeries, while the other serves as a catheterization laboratory. The BNC team conducted online meetings with Assistant Professor Hossam Al-Jehani, a highly qualified neurosurgeon with extensive experience in open vascular, neuro-endovascular, and neuro-critical care, before initiating the interventional procedures for the enrolled patients. Dr. Al-Jehani is situated in Dammam, Saudi Arabia, which is situated 944 kilometers (587 miles) from Baghdad. These meetings facilitated exhaustive discussions about the treatment strategies and the specific type of intervention that each patient required. The discussions were founded on a comprehensive examination of the patient's diagnostic images, which included computed tomography (CT) scans, CT angiography, magnetic resonance imaging (MRI), and catheter angiography. It is crucial to emphasize that the decision-making process and the implementation of teleproctoring were communicated to all selected patients as part of their treatment journey. The teleproctoring process commenced with the establishment of an efficient online connection between the angiography laboratory in Baghdad, Iraq, and the proctor in the KSA, using the Zoom application. A selected member of the BNC team was responsible for securely holding a phone affixed to a stand within the angiography suite. This arrangement allowed the proctor to remotely evaluate and supervise the pre-procedural preparations and offer assistance as required, both before and during the procedure. Occasionally, it was necessary to relocate to the angiography station during the procedure to engage in discussions with the proctor regarding decisions related to the initial contrast runs. Additionally, the proctor provided the surgical team with significant guidance and advice throughout the procedure, which facilitated ongoing discussions. As the surgeon approached critical stages and neared the finalization of the intervention, the discussions increased and were of greater importance.

Who is Dr. Hossam Al-Jehani?

Dr. Hosam Al-Jehani enrolled at Dammam University in 2002 and received a scholarship to pursue his education at McGill University in Montreal, Canada. There, he obtained the Royal College of Surgeons of Canada Fellowship in Neurosurgery. After that, he pursued a specialist fellowship in Neurocritical care. Furthermore, he successfully acquired a dual fellowship in cerebrovascular neurosurgery and interventional neuroradiology from McGill University and the University of Montreal. His scientific interests mostly revolve around understanding neural stem cells and their role in both normal development and pathological settings, such as intracerebral hemorrhages and traumatic brain damage. He resumed his position at the University of Dammam as an assistant professor and consultant specializing in neurosurgery, interventional neuroradiology, and

Neurocritical care. Additionally, he contributed to the advancement of the research field by publishing more than 100 research papers in prestigious journals on innovative subjects.

Outcomes of Baghdad-KSA collaboration

Neuro-endovascular procedures were meticulously selected for a total of seven cases that exhibited a variety of intracranial vascular lesions, spanning from July 2021 to March 2022. The patients' ages ranged from 26 to 48 years old. There were a variety of lesions, including two cases of brain arteriovenous malformation (AVM). One of the patients required two phases of embolization for their AVMs. In addition, there were two instances of supraclinoid internal carotid artery (ICA) aneurysms, one of Dura arteriovenous fistula, and the final case involved the preoperative embolization of a meningioma. It is crucial to note that none of the patients encountered any complications during or after the procedure. Every decision the proctor makes, or suggestion they make throughout the process is seen as constant stress from their perspective. Additionally, the proctor experiences a very difficult psychological condition as a result of the pressure to comprehend every element to make the best decision possible. It's the inner fear of what might happen if anything goes wrong. The technical difficulties of carrying out the entire interventional operation were present, but the surgical team was competent and could complete it. The majority of the proctoring attention was on cognitive and decision-making processes. Even if everything goes according to plan, there will still be stress on the proctor's part. Preparing for such proctoring in Iraq presented a difficult ethical issue and necessitated unusual pre-procedural contact with the patients. As a foreign physician consults with the surgical team and participates in their care, the patients in Iraq could have to deal with social issues. However, every patient understood that a Saudi Arabian associate professor would be collaborating virtually with the case team. Such precise patient permission is intriguing because online proctoring is not commonly used in Iraqi healthcare delivery. Moreover, their approval signifies their confidence in the medical professionals handling their cases.

Role of Mentees Within Baghdad-KSA Collaboration Program

In LMIC, including Iraq, there is a substantial need for proctoring services. Our teleproctoring experience, which utilizes common technology and promotes effective communication between the surgical team and the proctor, has shown its capacity to improve the learning experience for everyone involved and produce favorable results for patients in areas with limited resources. The mentees in the Baghdad-KSA collaboration program have played an indispensable role, significantly contributing to the program's success while simultaneously gaining invaluable experience. These mentees, who included residents, medical students, and junior surgeons, were actively involved in all phases of the teleproctoring sessions. From the outset, they engaged in preoperative planning discussions, where they were encouraged to ask questions and offer their insights on case management. This collaborative environment nurtured a sense of ownership and responsibility among the mentees, driving them to thoroughly understand the intricate details of each case.

During the course of the actual procedures, the mentees are not there just to passively watch; they participate. Under a remote proctor and direct supervision of senior surgeons, mentees have participated in selecting and preparing devices for use, with active contributions to the performance of critical decisions. This hands-on involvement exposed them to the most advanced neurointerventional devices and procedures, many of which were hitherto out of reach due to resource limitations in their home institutions. One of the most profound impacts of the teleproctoring experience on the mentees was the development of their technical skills. By following the detailed step-by-step guidance provided during the live-streamed procedures, mentees gained practical knowledge on how to navigate complex anatomical challenges, manage intraoperative complications, and apply advanced techniques such as coil embolization and flow diversion. The proctor's real-time feedback was invaluable, helping the mentees refine their techniques, improve their precision, and build their confidence in handling sophisticated neurovascular interventions. Beyond technical expertise, the teleproctoring experience also exerted character and professional attitude change on the mentees. Working at so high a level in which decisions must be so exact and quick required them to develop high situational awareness. Resiliency and mental quickness had to be developed due to this high level of demand for critical thinking and quick adaptations to unforeseen challenges. The collaborative nature of teleproctoring sessions, evidenced by constant communication with consequent feedback between the local surgical team and the proctor, further underlined the importance of teamwork and interprofessional collaboration to achieve optimum patient outcomes.

Finally, it is the neurointerventional aspects, ethical considerations at stake, and patient-centered approach to the same procedures that the mentees more appraised. The review of the outcomes,

complications, and follow-up plans for the patients in the postoperative reflection sessions impressed on them even more about the essence of continuous learning and meticulousness in patient care. These reflections assisted the mentees in respecting the broader implications of their occupations, culminating in a promise for continuous professional development and dedication to professional principles about healthcare standards in practice for community uplifting. Additionally, working in this international collaboration opened the mentees' eyes to various medical cultures and practices, hence broadening their perspectives. They learned to further appreciate the value of various approaches to problem-solving and how technology holds huge potential in bridging gaps between education and healthcare delivery. This increased their medical knowledge but also inspired them to look at neurosurgery from a global perspective and seek to contribute to its advancement at this level. Thus, the mentees who graduated from the Baghdad-KSA collaboration program emerged as more confident and forward-looking practitioners than their counterparts who had undergone the conventional training process. Now, they are better placed to tackle complex cases independently and mentor future generations on their own merit. Indeed, their growth testifies to the potential of teleproctoring programs in empowering healthcare professionals and effecting a change in the standard of care within resource-limited regions.
This experience also brought out that mentees have the potential to become leaders in their field and lead positive change within healthcare systems. Participating in this program has built technical skills but has also endowed them with critical thinking, communication, and leadership abilities necessary to navigate challenges in modern neurosurgery within a globalized world.

Challenges of Teleproctoring

High image quality for the remote proctor is essential in the context of online proctoring neurointerventional cases. In contrast to surgeries that prioritize the direct visualization of relatively large structures using fiber-optic cameras or microscopy, image-guided interventions present a distinctive set of obstacles. On the other hand, in neurointervention, the ongoing interpretation of dynamic angiographic image data of structures with limited visibility requires a proctor to acquire a real-time, high-level visualization of the operator's field of view. The primary components of this discipline are procedural techniques and the visualization of image data. As a result, the appropriate technologies were employed to transmit the field view to the proctor. Nevertheless, it is unnecessary to employ the sophisticated technology of videovisual image processing in order to establish the connection. The functionality of online proctoring is not contingent upon the most recent devices or sophisticated internet networks. In each of our instances, a basic mobile smartphone, a monthly subscription to the Zoom application, and a 4G internet connection were sufficient. Consequently, the effectiveness of such communication may be achieved through the use of basic and common devices.

Another logistical challenge for live-streaming was the time zone differences. Our experience was not affected by this issue as a result of the equivalent time zone between Iraq and the Kingdom of Saudi Arabia. The fitting of the headset onto surgical loupes was another prospective consideration. The surgeon's ability to utilize the headset may be impeded by the use of surgical loupes, which are employed in the majority of reconstructive surgical procedures, depending on the style of the loupes. We were able to engage in direct conversation without the use of a headset in our experience, as we had established an exceptionally calm environment prior to the operation. Situational awareness is considered a critical non-technical component of decision-making, in addition to technical issues. It can be implemented in complex medical procedures as a prerequisite for preventing complications. One of the objectives of the proctoring in our cases was to enhance awareness by utilizing basic technologies and visual video streaming.

Another obstacle was the ethical dilemma associated with the preparation of such proctoring in Iraq, which necessitated unique communication with the patients before the procedures. The patients in Iraq may encounter a societal issue as an external doctor participates in their case and guides the surgical team. Nevertheless, all of the patients concurred that an assistant professor from Saudi Arabia would be present online with the team in the case. The patients' uncomplicated consent is intriguing, as online proctoring is not a common practice in Iraqi healthcare delivery. Additionally, their consent is indicative of their confidence in the physicians who supervise their cases.

The continuous tension that the proctor experiences in every decision or piece of advice they provide during the procedure is a significant challenge from the proctor's perspective. Moreover, the proctor undergoes a highly demanding psychological state as a result of the strain to comprehend all conceivable details to make the most informed decision. The internal apprehension of what might transpire is the source of this dread. However, even if all is proceeding smoothly, the same level of tension as a proctor will be experienced.

Lessons Learned from the Baghdad-KSA Teleproctoring Experience

This teleproctoring initiative between Baghdad and KSA in the field of neurointerventional surgery offers an excellent opportunity for bridging educational and resource gaps in a region with limited access to specialized medical training. Several key lessons were learned from this collaboration that can be applied to similar settings in the future.

1. **The power of telemedicine in resource-limited settings:** One of the most significant lessons from this experience is the powerful role telemedicine can play in enhancing healthcare delivery in resource-limited settings. By leveraging common technology such as video conferencing platforms and internet connectivity, the Baghdad-KSA program demonstrated that high-quality surgical education and patient care can be achieved even in areas where physical access to experts is challenging. The success of the teleproctoring sessions showed that geographical barriers need not hinder the transfer of knowledge and skills, allowing for real-time guidance and mentorship that directly improves patient outcomes.
2. **Active learning through participation:** The involvement of the mentees in the teleproctoring sessions visually underlined that active participation by the learner in the process of learning was an open-ended process, much against the assimilation of knowledge in passive hues traditionally aligned with didactic learning. It is indeed a hands-on type of approach to push this teleproctoring program for the mentees right into the surgical procedures. This kind of active involvement at every step not only accelerated technical skill development but also deepened their understanding of complex neurointerventional techniques. It, therefore, emphasized that in medical education, one requires experiential learning whereby practice and real-time feedback are indispensable for the mastery of advanced procedures.
3. **Importance of collaboration and communication:** Requirements of teleproctoring sessions significantly contributed to the success of effective collaboration and communication. Key among them is seamless coordination between the local surgical team in Baghdad and the proctor in KSA so that each procedure is carried out with precision and care. Such experience shows the need for clear and constant communication, especially in high-stakes environments such as neurointerventional surgery. This collaboration was a

learning process in respect of developing one more important skill: long-distance communication, sharing of insights, and making decisions jointly. This is an important lesson in light of today's world, which is increasingly interconnected, having multidisciplinary and cross-border collaborations often seen in medical practice.

4. **Building resilience and adaptability:** The teleproctoring experience also taught valuable lessons in resilience and adaptability. Operating in a resource-limited environment with constraints on available equipment and materials required the surgical team and mentees to be flexible and resourceful. The need to adapt to the tools at hand and modify techniques accordingly reinforced the importance of being able to think on one's feet and find solutions to unexpected challenges. This adaptability is a critical skill for any surgeon, particularly in settings where ideal conditions are not always available.
5. **The ethical dimensions of remote proctoring:** There were ethical considerations in this teleproctoring experience. It was indispensable to engage patients in decision-making and obtain informed consent for procedures involving remote proctoring. The program thus impressed on the need for observing ethical standards in telemedicine, where the patients need full awareness of how their treatment is handled and relayed to an external expert. This lesson also emphasizes the clear communication and responsibility that are connected to the delivery of remote healthcare services.
6. **The role of technology in expanding access to education:** The successful implementation of teleproctoring with basic technological tools demonstrated that cutting-edge devices are not always necessary to achieve effective results. The use of a simple smartphone, video conferencing software, and a stable internet connection was sufficient to provide high-quality remote mentorship. This lesson is particularly important for other low- and middle-income countries, where access to advanced technology may be limited. It suggests that with the right approach, even modest technological resources can be used to expand access to medical education and improve healthcare delivery.
7. **Impact on professional development:** Indeed, this teleproctoring experience yielded transformational changes in the mentees when it came to fostering technical skills and professional identity. The said program has imbued a sense of responsibility, confidence, and commitment to lifelong learning. This mentee-mentor collaboration thus taught them to look at complex cases more analytically and reflectively, fathoming their broader

implications on the level of patient outcomes and healthcare standards. The experience thus serves to prepare them well for future leadership efforts so that they might make a contribution toward the development of neurosurgery in respective regions and beyond.

8. **Value of mentorship in accelerating learning curves:** This experience in teleproctoring has only cemented the fact that mentorship is a critical ingredient in medical education. Mentorship by a vastly experienced proctor improved the surgical outcomes of patients and accelerated the learning curve of the local team. This has further given them confidence and self-competency in doing neurointervention procedures. The program indeed brought out that mentorship, even across long distances, can be an effective way of developing the next generation of medical professionals.

One of the major impacts learned from this Baghdad-KSA collaboration would signal and prove, in a worthwhile manner, how teleproctoring and other programs raise medical education and patient care in places with resource limitations. Applied with technology, collaboration, and ethical standards, it will leave a mark on healthcare professionals and the communities they serve.

References

1. Sachdeva AK. Preceptoring, proctoring, mentoring, and coaching in surgery. Journal of Surgical Oncology. 2021 Oct;124(5):711-21.
2. Marosfoi M, Patel NV, Coon AL, Wald C, Repucci N, Nicholson P, Pereira VM, Wakhloo AK. International teleproctoring in neurointerventional surgery and its potential impact on clinical trials in the era of COVID-19: legal and technical considerations. Journal of NeuroInterventional Surgery. 2021 Nov 1;13(11):1022-6.
3. Hanning U, Bechstein M, Kaesmacher J, Boulouis G, Chapot R, Andersson T, Boccardi E, Psychogios M, Cognard C, de Dios Lascuevas M, Rodrigues M. Remote training of neurointerventions by audiovisual streaming: experiences from the European ESMINT-EYMINT E-fellowship program. Clinical neuroradiology. 2023 Mar;33(1):137-45.
4. Ismail M, Muthana A, Al-Ageely TA, Ahmed FO, Al-Taie RH, Al-Khafaji AO, Al-Zaidy MF, Salih HR, Alrawi MA, Aktham A, Al-Jehani H. Teleproctoring in therapeutic neurointervention: Experience from Iraq-Saudi Arabia collaboration. Surgical Neurology International. 2024;15.

Section 2: Collaborative and Research Initiatives

CH.8: Research Achievements of Mentees through Guided Mentorship and Publication Support

Rania H. Al-Taie, Saja Amer Albanaa, Mahmood F. Al-Zaidy, Mohammed A. Al-Dhahir, Teeba A. Al-Ageely, Samer S. Hoz

Section 2: Collaborative and Research Initiatives

CH.8: Research Achievements of Mentees through Guided Mentorship and Publication Support

Mentorship in academic medicine is the keystone of the development of research competencies and professional growth for young scientists and healthcare professionals. Good mentorship not only promotes technical skills but also enhances critical thinking, ethical considerations, and a collaborative approach toward research. In an increasingly complicated matter like healthcare, there cannot be enough appreciation for the role of mentorship in guiding mentees through such intricate landscapes of medical research. [1,2]. Research has consistently shown that mentorship significantly improves research productivity, quality, and impact. Mentees who receive high-quality mentorship are more likely to produce publishable research, secure funding, and advance in their academic careers. Moreover, mentorship contributes to higher job satisfaction and academic success, which are crucial for retaining talent within academic medicine [3,4]. The mentors provide an avenue for the mentees to develop confidence in their abilities to conduct independent research and acquire technical expertise. Programs with great emphasis on mentoring improve critical thinking, methodological rigor, and the ability to communicate research findings effectively. These are skills needed in the production of quality research likely to change practice or contribute meaningfully to the scientific community [2].

In addition to fostering personal and professional growth, mentorship also serves as a catalyst for innovation. Mentors help mentees navigate the challenges of research, encouraging them to explore new ideas and methodologies. This collaborative environment often leads to groundbreaking discoveries and innovative solutions to complex medical problems [5].

The examples in this chapter illustrate the dramatic impact mentorship can have on research results. Mentorship has not only allowed young researchers to provide valuable insight into their respective research areas but has also helped them grow into confident, independent professionals. These successes, driven by mentorship, underscore the continued investment in mentorship programs within academic medicine.

Mentorship-Driven Excellence in Neurosurgery Research

Mentorship in addressing traumatic brain injuries

Title: Blast-Induced Traumatic Brain Injuries: Experience from the Deadliest Double Suicide Bombing Attack in Iraq [6].

The traumatic brain injuries (TBIs), in relation to the complexity of the case and mostly the low level of resources in most areas prone to conflict, are a significant challenge. A research team led by their mentor, Dr. Hoz, finished an extensive study about patients with blast-induced traumatic brain injury with emphasis on outcomes from one of the deadliest double suicide bombings that happened in Iraq. The mentor played a crucial role in guiding his mentees through every stage of this challenging research project. From data collection in a high-stress environment to the analysis and interpretation of complex injury patterns, the mentorship ensured that the mentees understood the nuances of trauma research, including the ethical considerations involved in working with patients from conflict zones.

The paper that followed contributed valuable insight into the management of TBIs in conflict zones and has provided a benchmark against which future efforts would be gauged. For these mentees, research expertise acquired through the handling of sensitive data, carrying out rigorous analyses, and executing the publishing of high-impact research was an instructional methodology with a price tag that was beyond what these junior researchers could afford. Many have since gone on to further research in neurotrauma, for whom this project was a cornerstone for academic development.

Collaborative Research in Vascular Neurosurgery

Title: The Crux of Helix Curvature: Identifying a Potential Surface Landmark for the Anterior Border of the Sigmoid Sinus [7].

A critical component of neurosurgical procedures is that of identifying critical anatomical landmarks safely and effectively. In this respect, the mentor and his colleagues designed their study to find out the reliability of the surface landmark for the anterior border of the sigmoid sinus, representing an important area in minimally invasive neurosurgery. His mentorship was an instrumental factor in the completion of this multidisciplinary research project. He allowed his mentees to bring together different perspectives and approaches—from very detailed anatomical studies down to applying the findings to clinical practice. What he emphasized in his approach was collaborative effort, critical thinking, and rigorous validation of research findings.

The study resulted in a significant anatomical discovery that has implications for improving the safety and accuracy of neurosurgical procedures. The mentees involved in this project gained experience in multidisciplinary research, learning how to effectively collaborate with experts from various fields within the mentorship. The publication has been recognized for its contribution to neurosurgical practice and has opened new avenues for research in anatomical landmarks.

Mentorship in managing intraoperative challenges

Title: Management of Brain Aneurysm Neck-Avulsion During Clipping Surgery: An Illustrative Case and Literature Review [8].

Intraoperative rupture (IOR) is still among the most demanding complications neurosurgeons are called to face and, in most instances, defines the surgical outcome and prognosis for the patient. Avulsion of the brain aneurysm neck during clipping surgery is one type of IOR that is very difficult to manage and might very likely result in serious ischemic injury if not properly managed. A team of mentees investigated this subject. The mentor played a critical role in guiding his mentees, the co-authors of this study. They were medical students and junior doctors who worked on the project from literature review to the assessment and development of surgical techniques, all the way through to writing up a case report. The attending neurosurgeon was always there to advise me on that thin line between clinical practice and research so that the results were both academically sound and relevant for practical application. He also emphasized the importance of interdisciplinary collaboration, as the study involved not only neurosurgery but also radiology and critical care. His mentorship extended beyond the technical aspects, focusing on developing the mentees' ability to critically evaluate existing literature, synthesize new information, and apply it effectively in a clinical setting.

The surgical techniques for aneurysm neck-avulsion management, like the cotton-clip method, micro-suturing, and temporary clips, were discussed in detail in the paper. To that extent, the illustrative case was an application in real life and contributed some useful knowledge in the related area. It has given good experience in research work and clinical practice to the mentees in managing one of the major complications of vascular neurosurgery. The publication has been recognized for its contribution to the understanding and management of IOR in aneurysm surgery, and the mentees involved have been empowered to pursue further research and specialization in neurosurgery, equipped with the knowledge and confidence gained under Dr. Hoz's mentorship.

Addressing configurational changes in ruptured aneurysms through Multidisciplinary collaboration

Title: Configurational Changes of Ruptured Intracranial Aneurysms at the Window Between Pre-operative CTA and Definite Clipping Surgery [9].

Ruptured intracranial aneurysms are difficult neurosurgical cases. They become even more difficult when the aneurysms change during the time period between the first image at presentation and surgical intervention. Their changes complicate surgical procedures and may raise the risk of possible complications that arise during surgery. In this regard, in a study led by their mentor, changes were analyzed through a comparison of pre-operative CT angiography against intraoperative findings. The mentor provided invaluable guidance in such a complex research project using a multidisciplinary team composed of neurosurgeons, radiologists, and medical students. He was always insistent that there must be a collaboration between these specialties to get an appropriate evaluation done for pre-operative and intraoperative conditions of aneurysms. The mentor supplied his mentees with skills for assessing advanced imaging techniques that help understand the implications of the changes at the aneurysm, all aimed at improving surgical outcomes. Under his mentorship, the team developed a comprehensive methodology to retrospectively analyze cases of ruptured aneurysms, assessing the configurational changes that occurred between pre-operative imaging and surgery. The mentor's guidance ensured that the study was not only methodologically sound but also clinically relevant, providing actionable insights that could directly impact surgical practices.

The configurational changes had major impacts on the surgical approach and patient outcomes for some of the aneurysms. It further supported the close monitoring and potential requirement for re-imaging even in days immediately antecedent to surgery, especially if these delays cannot be avoided. Mentees involved with this project gain tremendous hands-on experience both in radiology and neurosurgery concerning data integration from multiple disciplines toward the optimization of patient care. The findings were published in the Romanian Neurosurgery journal, contributing to the broader understanding of aneurysmal behavior and its implications for surgical intervention. The collaborative nature of the research, guided by the mentor, demonstrated the importance of multidisciplinary approaches in tackling complex medical challenges, ultimately leading to improved patient outcomes and enhanced professional development for the mentees involved.

Exploring the psychosocial impact of neurosurgical interventions

Title: Till Death Do Us Part? The Inconspicuous Impact of Subarachnoid Haemorrhage on Conjugal Status [10].

Although it is life-threatening, a subarachnoid hemorrhage (SAH) has devastating physical effects but also serious psychological effects and social-relational consequences for the patient. The mentor who led this study discussed some of the truly overlooked effects of SAH on marital status and gave insights into the psychosocial aftermath of this neurological event. He guided a multidisciplinary team of neurosurgeons, neuropsychologists, and social scientists in traversing the complexities involved in studying the interface between medical outcomes and social dynamics. It was through his mentorship that a study could be designed to go beyond conventional metrics of medicine in an attempt to understand the broader implications for the lives of patients with SAH. The mentor emphasized the importance of understanding the holistic impact of medical interventions, encouraging his mentees to consider how physical health, cognitive function, and emotional well-being are interconnected. Under his guidance, the team conducted a comprehensive analysis that included both clinical data and qualitative assessments of patients' conjugal relationships after experiencing SAH.

The study had some very exciting findings about changes in conjugal relationships post-SAH. Although on one hand these relationships were found to deteriorate due to decreased cognitive abilities, personality changes, and physical dependence, on the other hand, some improved quite surprisingly, often due to a new appreciation for life and partnership from both parties, consequent to the near-fatal event. The publication highlighted the need for healthcare providers to consider the psychosocial dimensions of recovery in patients with SAH, advocating for integrated care approaches that address both the physical and emotional needs of patients. The mentees involved in this project gained valuable experience in conducting multidisciplinary research that bridges the gap between clinical practice and patient quality of life.

Collaborative management of complex spinal cord injuries

Title: Brown-Sequard Syndrome Associated with a Spinal Cord Injury Caused by a Retained Screwdriver: A Case Report and Literature Review [11].

Brown-Sequard Syndrome(BSS) is a neurological condition that results from hemisection of the spinal cord, commonly due to traumatic injuries. Diagnosis and management can be very challenging with retained foreign objects like screwdrivers. This case study described a 37-year-old male patient who suffered a spinal injury from the retained screwdriver, leading to BSS. He managed an interdisciplinary team, including neurosurgeons, emergency medicine specialists, and radiologists. His guide was very important in managing this case from diagnosis to surgical treatment. The mentor stressed the absolute need for an integrated approach whereby all members considered every aspect of patient care: further neurological deterioration risks, infection, and technical challenges unrelated to taking out an object. Under the mentorship, the team conducted a comprehensive literature review to compare the presented case with other instances of non-missile penetrating spinal injuries (NMPSIs). This involved analyzing the outcomes of similar injuries and discussing the best practices for managing such cases. The mentor's leadership in this project provided his mentees with valuable experience in both clinical decision-making and academic research, particularly in the context of rare and challenging medical conditions.

The study described the surgical management of the retained screwdriver, in which careful withdrawal of the object under direct vision was carried out to avoid further neurological damage. Postoperative outcomes were good, with significant improvement in motor function of the patient documented, although there was persistence in sensory deficits. This was further nailed with the publication of the article in Surgical Neurology International, which cemented global understanding of BSS secondary to retained foreign objects and provided insights into the best ways of managing such. Mentees involved in this research learned techniques for the management of complex spinal injuries and multidisciplinary collaboration for successful outcomes on the same. This case report, with its literature review, has since been referenced in similar cases—a tribute to how mentorship helped advance neurosurgery.

Managing complex penetrating brain injuries through multidisciplinary collaboration

Title: Transbasal Penetrating Traumatic Brain Injury Caused by a Rifle Rod: A Case Report [12].

Penetrating traumatic brain injuries (TBIs) represents a rare form of TBI and is surgically challenging, especially when the object involves unconventional ones. This case report, described by Dr. Samer S. Hoz, delineates complex management for a patient with a transbasal penetrating TBI from a rifle rod injury and depicts how multidisciplinary approaches play a role in achieving a positive outcome. Dr. Hoz also mentored the team, which was made up of neurosurgeons, otolaryngologists, and maxillofacial surgeons, among others, in handling this very rare and complicated case. His mentorship included how to navigate the sensitivities regarding the amalgamation of interdisciplinary expertise in the quest to develop a comprehensive surgical plan. He did this by guiding the team through the whole process, starting from degree imaging to the surgical extraction of the foreign body and post-operative care. He emphasized the need for precise preoperative planning and careful intraoperative management to avoid complications such as infection, cerebrospinal fluid leakage, and vascular injury. The mentor leadership ensured that each team member understood their role and worked collaboratively to achieve the best possible outcome for the patient.

The rifle rod was removed transnasally by the surgical team with the help of specialists in maxillofacial and otolaryngology. The postoperative course of the patient was uneventful; he recovered fully without neurological deficits. This case report that appeared in Surgical Neurology International gave key insights into the management of low-velocity penetrating TBIs, especially regarding the role of multidisciplinary management in such cases. The mentees involved in this project gained significant experience in managing complex traumatic injuries and learned the value of collaboration across specialties. The success of this case reinforced the importance of multidisciplinary teamwork in neurosurgery and demonstrated how mentors can effectively guide teams through the challenges of innovative surgical interventions.

Empowering medical students in neurosurgery

Title: Academic Productivity of Iraqi Medical Students in the Field of Neurosurgery: A Literature Review [13].

Despite huge challenges, such as limited resources and the impact of conflict, there has been an apparent surge in academic productivity within neurosurgery in Iraq, particularly in the realm of medical education. This paper by Dr. Hoz and colleagues overviewed the recent years of academic contribution of Iraqi undergraduate medical students in neurosurgical science. The paper contributes to the idea that mentorship plays a critical role in bringing out research and professional growth among students. Dr. Hoz has led in the mentorship of Iraqi medical students, particularly in the difficult times of COVID-19, for research and provision of guidelines to improve academic production from these students. His mentorship program, entitled the "Baghdad Neurosurgery Mentorship," resulted in engaging more than 500 students, most of whom got the chance to be involved in real-time neurosurgical operations and research projects. This mentorship extended beyond just academic instruction; he focused on developing the student's research skills, critical thinking, and ability to adapt to a rapidly changing environment. His guidance helped students navigate the complexities of publishing in international journals despite the obstacles posed by Iraq's academic infrastructure.

The review indicated that between January 2020 and December 2022, 47 Iraqi medical students from various universities contributed to 60 international neurosurgical publications. The increased academic productivity of these students is directly related to structured mentorship, empowering students to develop meaningful research. This even involves first-time authors whose resumes have been significantly augmented by their involvement in impactful studies, hence improving their chances for further studies and jobs. The impact of the mentor is evident not only in the increased number of publications but also in the quality of research produced. His approach has set a new standard for medical education in Iraq, demonstrating that with the right guidance and support, students can overcome significant barriers to achieving academic success.

Developing research skills through mentorship

Title: Reinvigorating Medical Student Mentorships in Neurosurgery During the Pandemic: Lessons Learned from Iraq [14].

Challenges posed by the COVID-19 pandemic to medical education are unique worldwide. In Iraq, the situation was still complicated by existing infrastructural weaknesses. However, the mentor used this period as an opportunity to reinvigorate mentorship in neurosurgery. This paper shares some of the methods and outcomes of mentorship initiatives adopted during the pandemic. It is under the initiatives of the mentor, Dr. Hoz, that online mentorship programs have been driven, enabling medical students to continue their education and research activities despite restrictions. Such mentorship truly characterized flexibility and innovation in mentorship: workshops, seminars, one-on-one mentoring sessions, everything was conducted via digital platforms. These programs equip students with the ability to conduct independent research, analyzing data and publishing the findings, now also in a remote setting. Students were encouraged to engage with ongoing research projects, resulting in a significant increase in publications. The mentor's efforts ensured that the disruption caused by the pandemic did not hinder the academic progress of his mentees but rather provided them with new tools and strategies to succeed in a challenging environment.

These activities of mentorship consequently increased the number of research publications by Iraqi medical students during the pandemic. The skills and confidence built up through these programs contributed to a long-lasting effect whereby many of the students continued their research careers and made important contributions to Neurosurgery in Iraq and internationally.

Co-Authored Neurosurgical Books as a Mentorship Legacy

First of all, when I think about books and chapters that I've had the privilege to write or contribute to, I don't perceive these as my works alone. Sure, I see more than that. I see a collaboration of effort between myself and the mentees working tirelessly for this very purpose: pushing the boundaries of neurosurgical knowledge further. These publications are just as much an outcome of their intense labor and committed efforts as they were mine.

- **Vascular Neurosurgery in Multiple-Choice Questions:** One of the projects that really stands out is Vascular Neurosurgery: In Multiple-Choice Questions. This book has been a crucial resource for those preparing for the American Board of Neurosurgery exams. But what truly makes this book special is the role the mentees played in its creation. The mentor guided them through the research process, but it was their fresh perspectives and curiosity that brought new insights into the material. This project wasn't just about publishing a book; it was about building their confidence and expertise, giving them a platform to contribute to the field in a meaningful way.
- **Neurotrauma in Multiple-Choice Questions:** This book is a collective effort; the mentees were deeply involved in creating case studies and questions that form the core of this book. Working closely, they analyzed complex neurotrauma cases, and they learned how to use critical thinking skills in their approaches to challenges for both the OR and academic publishing. I remember watching those who began as students grow to co-authors during this process—it is one of the more rewarding experiences in my career.

- **Pineal Neurosurgery:** It is another example of the significant roles that the mentees took on in this. They got involved in all the intricate details of pineal region tumours. They participated in getting the newest research, writing sections of the book, and even participating in the rigorous process of case reviews. This wasn't them contributing to a book, this was mastering complex subspecialty knowledge which would help set them apart in their careers.
- **Neurosurgery Board Favorites, Crossword Puzzles:** The mentees were instrumental in this project, designing puzzles that were both challenging and educational. They brought creativity and a deep understanding of neurosurgical concepts to the table. This project was a chance for them to explore how education can be engaging, and it's been incredible to see how well it's been received in the neurosurgical community.

Apart from these books, I have also had the opportunity to write chapters for some collective works, and there, my mentees have indeed been a part of the process. In the chapter in relation to Neurofibroma in Tumors and Cancers: Central and Peripheral Nervous Systems, for example, it became possible for my mentees and me to work through the pathology, diagnosis, and management of neurofibromas. This involved taking the lead in reviewing recent publications and drafting of content, thereby deepening neuro-oncology knowledge. Similarly, in the chapter on the Pathophysiology of Cerebral Aneurysms in Endovascular Surgery of Cerebral Aneurysms, we worked together to dissect the underlying mechanisms of cerebral aneurysms. My mentees were hands-on in every step, from literature review to writing, and this experience gave them a solid foundation in both the basic science and clinical aspects of aneurysms.

In attempting Mechanical Thrombectomy: Techniques and Devices in Neurointerventional Surgery: Current Status and Future Prospects, we worked as a team to be at the forefront of neurointerventional surgery. My mentees researched state-of-the-art techniques and devices and helped write a chapter that will not only inform others but also increase their own understanding of this extremely important procedure. Finally, contributing to the book Understanding and Managing Cerebral Aneurysms was another collaborative milestone. My mentees and I worked together to provide a comprehensive approach to diagnosing, treating, and managing cerebral aneurysms. This project was an incredible learning experience for them, giving them the opportunity to apply their research skills and contribute to a significant medical text.

These publications, books, and chapters are testament to the mentorship relationships that I have had the privilege of creating with my mentees. Such projects impart not only knowledge but also offer a view of the experience of contributing meaningfully to neurosurgical literature. My hope is that these experiences prepare them well enough to continue the legacy forward by advancing our field through research, teaching, or clinical practice. These works are our collective contribution to the future of neurosurgery.

Essential Lessons and Impact

The examples provided by in this chapter give insight into the transformational change that effective mentorship can bring about within the field of neurosurgery. The approach to mentorship represents one in which an interdisciplinary collaborative culture is being raised, with an emphasis on development in research and professional growth. One of the key lessons learned is the importance of a mentor who not only imparts technical knowledge but also instills confidence and a sense of responsibility in their mentees. Dr. Hoz's mentorship has consistently emphasized the importance of critical thinking, ethical considerations, and the application of research findings to real-world clinical scenarios. His guidance has enabled his mentees to navigate complex medical challenges, resulting in successful publications that contribute to the broader field of neurosurgery. Another important takeaway is the mentor who stimulates innovation and adaptability. Whether it be in leading complex surgical procedures, performing multidisciplinary research, or simply adjusting to challenges such as COVID-19, the mentor has instilled in his mentees the ability to approach their work with contextual intelligence by always keeping in mind that there may be a better way to do things. This flexibility has not only helped to ensure his research results but also better prepared his mentees for facing the upcoming challenges in contemporary medicine.

The long-term impact of mentorship is evident in the continued success of his mentees, many of whom have gone on to become leaders in their own right. These individuals are now contributing to the field of neurosurgery not just as practitioners but also as researchers, educators, and mentors themselves. By perpetuating the cycle of knowledge and skill transfer initiated by the mentor, these former mentees are ensuring that the lessons they have learned are passed on to the next generation of neurosurgeons. This ripple effect of the mentorship is evident in the growing body of research his past mentees are producing, modern and creative clinical practices being opened, and mentorship programs they currently lead. It is within this perpetual cycle of mentorship and professional development that credence is lent to the enduring legacy left by the work of the mentor, solely through effective mentorship, therefore, it shapes a field's future, propels medical knowledge, and positively impacts health care worldwide.

In conclusion, the mentorship has not only resulted in a legacy of successful publications but has also fostered the development of competent, independent researchers who continue to push the boundaries of neurosurgery. His commitment to his mentees has created a foundation for continued innovation and excellence in the field, ensuring that his influence will be felt for generations to come.

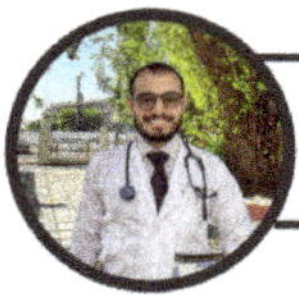

Ahmed Muthana

I attended medical school at a very opportune time when Dr. Hoz, an Iraqi pioneer in vascular neurosurgery, was doing yearly mentorship for medical students. Joining the Hoz mentorship in the fourth stage of medical school was a pivotal change in my life. Not only did it upgrade my scientific level in medicine, but also improved my personal growth and development in different aspects. My mentality shifted from being a complainer and procrastinator to being reasonable, responsible, and hard-working. I learned how small steps are crucial in achieving a bigger goal and how internal motivation is more powerful than seeking external support from others.

I still remember that day when Dr. Hoz called me at midnight while I was drawing a portrait. "*I'm sorry if the time is inappropriate,*" he said. "*Not at all, I'm already awake and drawing a portrait,*" I replied. He was amazed and said, "*That would be your secret weapon in your future career.*" This was my introduction to the field of medical illustration. I struggled at first because I was obligated to use digital drawing instead of paper. After watching many tutors and taking several courses, I finally was able to get used to this digital world of drawing. Although I did not set out to be a medical illustrator, my curiosity in both art and science was unveiled during and after the Hoz mentorship.

Dr. Hoz was in every step of this journey; he used to motivate, encourage, and guide me to develop a keen eye for detail and artistic precision. He always reviews and provides daily feedback about each illustration to make sure that the work is acceptable and perfect both artistically and scientifically.

Not only a medical illustrator, Dr. Hoz has gifted me with a researched mind. He showed me the right path to enter the research field and have a solid background in scientific research. Thanks to him, I now have 50+ published papers in different decent and respectful journals. I acquired experience in doing multiple types of research, from case reports to systematic reviews. We do monthly meetings to discuss different ideas about research projects, review multiple papers and author styles, and try to enhance our style in writing as much as we can.

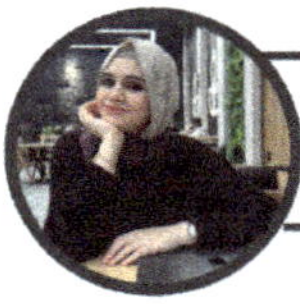

Sama Al-Bairmani

It is difficult to describe our experience with the most encouraging mentor anyone could ask for. Going back September 5, 2019, it all started when we first met at the HOZ lab in the neurosurgery teaching hospital in Baghd with the mentorship lasting for one month and followed by attending surgeries, writing research papers, chap contributions, and attending neurosurgical conferences for medical students as a one team. For me, joining mentorship as a first-year medical student, knowing nothing about the brain, was really challenging. Questions "How am I going to catch up with them? How am I going to understand these radiographs? From where I sho start?" were ringing in my head, but with a passionate caring mentor nothing is impossible.

During this time, I have participated in writing some research papers, but the first paper assigned to me as a f author was in 2022, which had a special taste. I still remember the day Dr. HOZ called me and told me that paper is going to be about a super advanced topic through which we are going to propose a new classification syst regarding a complex surgical approach. This paper was not just an addition to my scientific knowledge, but a represented a new challenge that added to my personal experience and made me eager to learn more that we star writing a second paper about the same topic but with more complex combined approaches as soon as we publis the first one! Now after six years of commitment to this challenging specialty, I am grateful that I have started journey since an early age. It changed my mind set and the way I think and perceive things, and it made me rea that medicine is not just about science and medical knowledge, but also about communication and teamwork, ab discussing ideas and thoughts out loud and benefit from colleagues and staff. Being in a community involve stude from different stages with varying experiences along the presence of a guiding mentor who listens to ev participant is a life changing experience. This mentorship made me realize that a great mentor is always present supportive, as Dr. HOZ was not with me just during the training in Baghdad, but he stood with me along ev academic step, including a clinical training program I took in the United Kingdom, Bristol. He was there whene I have a question of how to use my time perfectly during my presence in there, and I used to call him whenev needed help or wanted a better opinion.

We will always remember the first hand that took our hands and taught us how to be in an OR, the first one v guided us into a research writing opportunity while we're still in college, and the one who always trusted in eac us more than we trust ourselves.

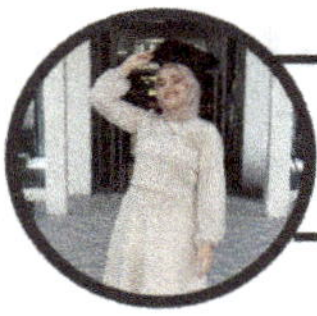

Abrar A. Khoailed

fore I got into medical school the only goal that I had was to "make a lifetime change for my patients" as I told mother back then, it was just a simple idea from the dreams of the young woman I was back then. Until some dom school day in my second year, I heard some of my friends talking about a mentorship which wasn't that resting until the word "neurosurgery" came into conversation because the only passion I could ever find in such r of medical school was in the lectures of the nervous system.

er the first meeting in the HOZ mentorship program, I knew - at that time - this was the answer to the young man's dream to make the forever-lasting change she always wanted, and after months of meetings I got the nce to get into my first operation theatre with the specialist - that I remember clearly till now - which was an 'OM aneurysm clipping surgery.

the initial training that was a part of this mentorship, I got the courage to tell my mentor dr. Hoz "I'm ready to dle a project from zero" to which he asked, "What topic do you prefer to be your project about", I simply wered "Vascular neurosurgery" as passion has drawn me back to that same first operation I ever witnessed.

the distracted person I was back then I decided one thing, I am always going to follow what I feel, so it started m writing a review about temporary clipping to the point of finishing a new book from scratch. He told me back n "This is the first time in the history of this mentorship that a junior medical student would start a neuroanatomy k by himself", so I had the confidence that my mentor's trust has recurrently built in me, and I did it with a lot collaborations with our amazing team.

w I am an editor and chapter author included in all chapters in the "Neuroanatomy board favorites crossword zle" book, and if you wonder what happened to the first project that I tried to complete, I got it published in the manian Neurosurgery under the title "Temporary clipping in intracranial aneurysm surgery. History and elopment".

first exposure - including the first neurosurgical operation I witnessed - turned into this applicable passion, and young woman found her way to work into her lifetime remarkable change as a doctor.
Hoz's mentorship was not just an inspiration to me but a chance for guidance to work on everything I dreamed ut. Finally, I learned to always follow my passion and do what my heart tells me to without any ounce of itation.

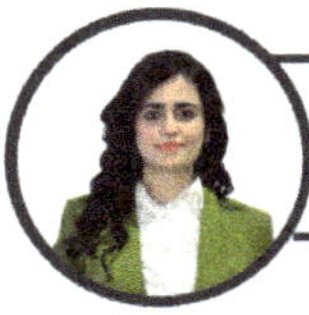

Noor M. Shaker

It's like you have the raw material inside your brain and power, passion, enthusiasm in your heart and you d know how channel it.

As a first-generation doctor, I faced many challenges. I had no support and no clear path to follow after I achi my goal of entering medical school. So, what's next? Life without goals is just wasted time.
I really needed a mentor to guide me, support me, acknowledge me, and believe in me as any new doctor als teach you attitude ethics to find my own way by myself, I didn't understand the true meaning of a mentor program which was what I need in that time.

That was until I was in my 4th year in medical school, I participated in an online meeting with Dr. Hoz. I inspiring honest wise person with others from different country and stages all gathered to meet with Dr.Hoz why? and how can it continues ? As a why I think every different person have a different answer. I asked Dr. how to stay involved, he told me that if I was interested and committed, the program was open to anyone wanted to pursue knowledge and scientific goals.
After that Dr.Hoz invited me to an operation day which consisted of staying from early morning for preparatior patient to operation and how to deal with patient with problem in his brain and his family to operation to operation till ward to be reasurence to the patient healthy

Later, I had the opportunity to join the team in writing a medical research paper, which was a dream come tru me. Research became a meditative space where I could channel my passion. It gave me the confidence I needed clarified my career goals.
This experience also inspired me to lead research discussions at my university, where I had the chance to exp what medical research is and whether it's something students can pursue during medical school. I was surprise learn that more than 90% of students don't know about medical research or mentorship programs, which made even more eager to spread this knowledge. During my time in the section, the dean of my college asked if I h doctor in my family, which made him wonder if I was a first-generation doctor. Thank you, Dr. Hoz, for hel me realize that, even without a medical family, I am supported in my journey. It's the mentorship and guid from incredible mentors like you that truly make a difference in achieving our medical goals."

The mentorship program with Dr. Hoz and his team helped me become more selfless, honest, and clear-heade I received two "official letter of thanks and appreciation" in addition to a gift from my university!
That was never given to anyone before. I am incredibly proud of this achievement, as it has made me better academically and personally.

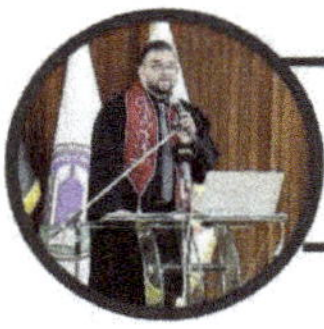

Ali. M. Neamah

›king back, the Hoz Neurosurgery Mentorship Program was a pivotal moment in my career, shaping the way I roach medicine, mentorship, and personal growth. In 2019, I had the privilege of both participating in and organizing program, marking my first real exposure to structured mentorship. Over the course of three weeks at the ırosurgical Teaching Hospital, we were immersed in an environment that not only shaped us as future doctors but as educators, researchers, and mentors for those who would follow in our footsteps. This program instilled in us a ng sense of discipline, teamwork, and continuous self-improvement, lessons that have stayed with me ever since.
ing this mentorship, I had the opportunity to deliver several lectures, including "How to Read Brain CT Scans" and ontaneous Subarachnoid Hemorrhage (SAH)," both aimed at equipping mentees with essential knowledge in roimaging and critical care. It is incredibly fulfilling to know that my Brain CT Scan lecture is still being used by dents today. This experience not only deepened my knowledge but also ignited my interest in medical education. litionally, I became involved in research projects that fueled my scientific curiosity and commitment to evidence-ed medicine.
ond the initial program, my involvement in mentorship continued as I delivered lectures both online and in-person ıbsequent programs. Through these opportunities, I gained a deeper understanding of the importance of mentorship ridging knowledge gaps and fostering professional development. Mentorship, I've realized, is a two-way street—le I guided others, I also refined my teaching skills and expanded my own understanding, especially when it came ıaking important career decisions.
of the most rewarding aspects of mentorship has been witnessing the lasting impact it has on others. Many mentees e shared how these sessions boosted their confidence and helped them navigate their professional paths. This firmed my belief that mentorship is not just about passing on knowledge but also about inspiring, supporting, and owering the next generation of medical professionals. It fosters a culture of lifelong learning and collaboration, ch is essential in the field of medicine.
reover, the program forged a lifelong bond among the participants. We became more than colleagues—we became mily. To this day, we continue to support one another, collaborating on research and academic projects. Many of us e gone on to organize and teach in subsequent mentorship programs, ensuring that the cycle of learning continues. s is the essence of mentorship—you begin as a mentee, become a mentor, and eventually guide the next generation. ough these experiences, I have grown not only as a mentor but also as a learner. Mentorship has taught me resilience, ptability, and the value of sharing knowledge. It has been an incredible journey—one that I hope to continue, tributing to the growth and development of future mentees while also evolving in my own career.

s mentorship program not only deepened our understanding of neurosurgery but also helped each of us discover t we truly wanted from medicine. It guided us in defining our path—whether as researchers, educators, or clinicians. program also helped us understand whether we had a medical or surgical mindset, shaping our awareness and urity in ways that extended far beyond academics.
ough this experience, I gained clarity about my specialty choice and learned to think outside the box, always nning not just the next step, but the five steps ahead. I discovered how to stand out, grow, and evolve—not by king alone, but by collaborating with a strong team. The program showed me that the right team can help you leap vard in ways that would take years if you were on your own.From that moment on, I made a commitment: to always ıre that those who come after me are even better than I was, because the stronger the team, the stronger I become.

pecial thank you to Dr. Samer Hoz for his dedication and efforts in making this mentorship program possible. His on and guidance have created a lasting impact on all of us who were fortunate to be part of this journey.

References

1. Sambunjak D, Straus SE, Marušić A. Mentoring in academic medicine: a systematic review. Jama. 2006 Sep 6;296(9):1103-15.
2. da Silva Souza RC, Bersaneti MD, dos Santos Yamaguti WP, Baia WR. Mentoring in research: Development of competencies for health professionals. BMC nursing. 2023 Jul 26;22(1):244.
3. Walensky RP, Kim Y, Chang Y, Porneala BC, Bristol MN, Armstrong K, Campbell EG. The impact of active mentorship: results from a survey of faculty in the Department of Medicine at Massachusetts General Hospital. BMC medical education. 2018 Dec;18:1-8.
4. Beck Dallaghan GL, Coe CL, Wright ST, Jordan SG. Mentoring medical education research: Guidelines from a narrative review. Medical Science Educator. 2022 Jun;32(3):723-31.
5. Toh RQ, Koh KK, Lua JK, Wong RS, Quah EL, Panda A, Ho CY, Lim NA, Ong YT, Chua KZ, Ng VW. The role of mentoring, supervision, coaching, teaching and instruction on professional identity formation: a systematic scoping review. BMC medical education. 2022 Jul 8;22(1):531.
6. Hoz SS, Al-Sharshahi ZF, Dolachee AA, Al-Smaysim AM, Matti WE, Bydon A, Kadhum HJ. Blast-induced traumatic brain injuries: experience from the deadliest double suicide bombing attack in Iraq. World neurosurgery. 2021 Jan 1;145:e192-201.
7. Hoz SS, Palmisciano P, Algburi HA, Sharma M, Ismail M, Andaluz N. The crux of helix curvature: A potential surface landmark for the anterior border of the sigmoid sinus in minimally invasive presigmoid approaches. Surgical Neurology International. 2022;13.
8. Al-Ageely TA, Ismail M, Alsaadi SB, Salim FF, Kareem ZM, Talib SH, Jaafer H, Hoz SS. Management of brain aneurysm neck-avulsion during clipping surgery: Illustrative case and literature review. Romanian Neurosurgery. 2023 Jun 15:164-9.
9. Algburi HA, Ismail M, Al-Nuaimi TM, Alzeyadi ZT, Sabbar JM, Al-Kishawi AK, Al-Taie RH, Al-Zaidy MF, Alrawi MA, Hoz SS. Configurational changes of ruptured intracranial

aneurysms at the window between pre-operative CTA and the definite clipping surgery. Romanian Neurosurgery. 2024 Jun 15:200-4.

10. Hoz SS, Alfawares Y, Ismail M, Al-Kishawi F, Andaluz N. Till death do us part? The inconspicuous impact of subarachnoid haemorrhage on conjugal status. Romanian Neurosurgery. 2023 Dec 15:419-22.
11. Abdulqader MN, Ismail M, Al-Khafaji AO, Al-Ageely TA, Kareem ZM, Al-Baider RA, Albairmani SS, Ayad F, Hoz SS. Brown-Sequard syndrome associated with a spinal cord injury caused by a retained screwdriver: A case report and literature review. Surgical Neurology International. 2022;13.
12. Al-Alousi HM, Al-Kubaisi KT, Ismail M, Al-Ageely TA, Abdulameer AO, Aluaibi SA, Al-Taie RH, Hoz SS. Transbasal penetrating traumatic brain injury caused by a rifle rod: A case report. Surgical Neurology International. 2022;13.
13. Ismail M, Algburi HA, Al-Khazaal YM, Daily SK, Mohsin HE, Jaafar H, AbdulWahid J, Andaluz N, Hoz SS. Academic productivity of Iraqi medical students in the field of neurosurgery: A literature review. Surgical Neurology International. 2023;14.
14. Hoz SS, Ismail M, Almufadhal MH, Al-Ageely TA, Aljuboori Z. Reinvigorating medical student mentorships in neurosurgery during the pandemic: Lessons learned from Iraq. Surgical Neurology International. 2022;13.

Section 2: Collaborative and Research Initiatives

CH.9: Academic Participation of Mentees in Conferences, Seminars, and Scientific Forums

Rania H. Al-Taie, Bandar M. Al Hadeethi, Alkawthar M. Abdulsada, Mohammed S. Al-Baldawi, Teeba A. Al-Ageely

Section 2: Collaborative and Research Initiatives

CH.9: Academic Participation of Mentees in Conferences, Seminars, and Scientific Forums

To reach the highest level of achievement, a physician, and a neurosurgeon in particular, needs to go through five main levels to eventually be a world-class scientist. These levels are the personal level, the local institution level, the national level, the international level, and the world-class level. The main focus of the mentorship, which is reflected in the mentees' experiences, revolves around enhancing and achieving excellence on a personal level. This level draws attention to the basic individual characteristics and theoretical knowledge in the practical aspects. These basic personal characteristics include 2 main components: the knowledge and passion for learning and the clinical skills required in surgery in general and in neurosurgery in particular [13].

In the medical field, confidence accounts for a major part of an individual's success overall. Many medical students and young physicians face a lot of challenges that require confidence to solve. One of the methods that could establish confidence in medical students and build their self-esteem is exposure. For instance, the skill of public speaking is usually greatly solidified by practice; many individuals experience much more confidence after making a presentation, and their mistakes help them improve their performance during the next presentation.

In the demanding world of medicine, presentations serve as both a rite of passage and a fundamental component of medical education. They are a platform where mentees demonstrate not only their knowledge but also their ability to communicate complex ideas with clarity and confidence. Presentations in a mentorship setting are particularly significant as they provide mentees with the opportunity to engage in deep learning, receive invaluable feedback, and cultivate the professional attributes essential for their future careers. This chapter explores the multifaceted role of presentations within the medical mentorship model, offering guidance on how to maximize their educational value.

The Importance of Presentations in Medical Training

1. **Skill development**: There is much more to presentations in medical training than an exercise in public speaking. This represents an opportunity for mentorship for the mentee to develop important skills, broadly speaking. For example, identifying a large body of information composed of complicated medical material and synthesizing it into one clear, cohesive narrative is a skill developed through regular presentations. This process requires mentees to be critically reflective about their learning, put their thoughts together logically, and detect in advance what the audience may require. The presentation helps to actually develop a mentee's ability to interpret information at hand and further relay it at appropriate levels. Presentation given to appreciate patient cases can either make or break the situation in clinics; proper presentation will determine the course of treatment a patient gets. For example, in the context of a case presentation for a multidisciplinary team, the clarity with which information is relayed may serve to affect the direction of diagnosis and treatment. [1].
2. **Knowledge consolidation**: The act of preparing for a presentation forces mentees to engage with their material in a deeper, more meaningful way. This process is critical for the consolidation of knowledge. When mentees prepare a presentation, they must thoroughly understand the content, anticipate questions, and think critically about how best to convey the information. This level of engagement reinforces their learning and aids in the retention of information, making it more accessible for future clinical application. In particular, case presentations require the mentee to integrate knowledge from various disciplines, apply clinical reasoning, and demonstrate their understanding of the patient's condition. This integration of knowledge is essential for the development of a well-rounded medical professional. Furthermore, research presentations, where mentees present findings from their scientific investigations, also contribute significantly to knowledge consolidation. These presentations not only deepen the mentee's understanding of the research process but also reinforce the scientific principles that underpin clinical practice [2].
3. **Feedback mechanism**: It is one of the cornerstone foundational concepts of medical education, as presentations provide an organized opportunity for this from mentors. A

mentor could then provide detailed feedback after having made a presentation that would be immediate and specific, indicating areas of strengths while at the same time pointing out opportunities for improvement. This kind of feedback assists in furthering the mentee's growth in that it will outline for him or her where he/she is strong and where to put more emphasis on effort [1]. Constructive feedback is not just about correcting mistakes; it's about guiding mentees toward developing better clinical reasoning, refining their communication style, and encouraging them to reflect on their performance. For example, a mentor might point out that while the content of a presentation was solid, the delivery lacked engagement and suggested techniques to improve this aspect. Such insights are invaluable as they help mentees to build confidence and become more effective communicators.

4. **Professionalism**: This process of preparation and delivery of presentations teaches the mentee professionalism in every respect of their work. Professionalism in presentations is not only about the content itself but also about its presentation. It trains mentees to respect the time of those who have to listen to them, be brief, be ethical in presenting their work, give credit where credit is due, and handle criticism and questions with dignity and respect [3]. Furthermore, presentations often take place in formal settings, such as grand rounds or conferences, where mentees are observed by senior professionals. This setting provides a unique opportunity for them to practice professionalism in a real-world context, which includes dressing appropriately, using professional language, and adhering to the ethical standards of medical practice. These experiences are critical in preparing mentees for the professional responsibilities they will face throughout their careers.
5. **Networking:** For a medical student or even young residents, being under shed light gives them recognition and acknowledgment overall. This will allow for experiences of networking and making connections with people in similar specialties and interests, consequently facilitating possible collaborations in the future. Moreover, initiatives like this count as experience points that can add to one's resume.

Types of presentations in the Hoz Mentorship

There are generally three forms of presentations performed by mentees, each with precise benefits. These categories include case reports and case presentations, research presentations, and educational presentations.

- **Case presentations**: Case presentations are the signature to medical mentorship; the mentee prepares an opportunity to demonstrate their skills in clinical reasoning and decision-making. The mentee formally presents a patient's case from initial presentation through history, physical exam, workup, treatment plan, and follow-up. A case presentation requires the mentee to assimilate a plethora of information, identify what is pertinent, and then present this information in a logical, coherent manner.

Case presentations also offer an opportunity for mentees to receive feedback on their clinical reasoning. For example, a mentor might challenge the mentee's differential diagnosis or suggest alternative management strategies. These discussions are invaluable for the mentee's development, as they provide insight into the complexities of clinical decision-making and expose the mentee to different perspectives [4].

- **Research presentations**: Research presentations are considered paramount in academic medicine, especially for the dissemination and contribution of knowledge. Presentations to mentees are a great avenue for enhancing their capabilities in understanding research and how to present scientific findings. Well-presented research shows that a mentee can conduct rigorous research, analyze the data, and draw effective conclusions.

Research presentations also help mentees to engage with the broader medical community. Presenting at conferences or symposiums exposes mentees to new ideas, fosters collaboration, and allows them to receive feedback from experts in the field. These experiences are invaluable for mentees who aspire to have careers in academic medicine, as they provide a foundation for future research and scholarship [5].

- **Teaching presentations**: Teaching is a very important aspect of medical practice. Presentations are one form of developing teaching skills in mentees whereby there is a need to simplify complex medical ideas and explain to peers and junior trainees in clear, concise ways and with much flair. It thus pushes the mind of the mentee further into thinking critically about just how this information might best be relayed to the audience in an understandable way.

The ability to teach is a marker of deep understanding, and teaching presentations helps to reinforce the mentee's knowledge while also contributing to the education of others. These presentations are often interactive, with the mentee encouraging questions and discussions, which further enhances the learning experience for all involved [6].

Preparing for a Successful Presentation

One of the preliminary steps in preparing a successful presentation is to understand the audience. In developing a presentation, mentees need to take into consideration the level of knowledge, interests, and level of expectations from the audience. As an illustration, a case presentation for fellow students may focus more on the basics of diagnosis and treatment; inversely, a presentation to established clinicians might explore subtler aspects of differential diagnosis and advanced treatment options. In addition, a well-structured presentation is key to maintaining the audience's attention and conveying the intended message effectively. Mentees should begin with a clear introduction that outlines the objectives of the presentation, followed by the main content that is logically organized, and end with a conclusion that summarizes the key points. It is important for mentees to ensure that the content is clear, concise, and relevant, with complex ideas broken down into understandable segments. Moreover, the use of visual aids, such as slides, charts, and diagrams, can enhance the presentation. However, it is crucial that these visual aids are used judiciously and complement the spoken words rather than overwhelming the audience. Mentees should be trained on how to design effective visuals that highlight the key points of their presentation without distracting from the message.

Practice is key. In all aspects, practice is an important issue. Mentees should be advised to conduct several practices before their presentations with a mentor or a peer who has the allowance to give commentary. Such practice helps the mentees to refine their delivery, manage their timing, and develop confidence. Practicing also gives room for one to identify and solve possible hitches before the actual presentation [7]. Time management is another important feature in the preparation. Most mentees have difficulties keeping their presentations within the proposed limits. Practice with a timer will let them get a good sense of pacing in the presentation and make sure that they include all the necessary points, but not over the specified time.

Common Challenges and Solutions

It is quite normal that the mentees may feel apprehensive prior to a presentation in front of a large or senior audience. Sometimes, this nervousness does interfere with their actual performance. The mentor should motivate the mentees to practice extensively, rehearsing in front of small groups so that they build up their capability. Deep breathing, positive visualization, and mindfulness might also help reduce anxiety.

Managing time effectively during a presentation is a common challenge for many mentees. Mentors should emphasize the importance of practicing with a timer and planning the presentation to ensure that it fits within the allotted time. It may also be helpful to advise mentees to prepare a condensed version of their presentation in case they need to shorten it on the fly.

The mentees might be intimidated by difficult or unexpected questions. Train the mentees on how to prepare for any possible questions and how to respond in instances where they do not know something right off the bat. Mentees need to be taught it is okay to say they do not know, and they certainly can tell them that they can find out the answer and get back to them later [8].

The Role of Mentors in Mentees' Presentations

The mentor's role in the preparation phase is critical. Mentors should provide support and guidance on how to choose appropriate topics, structure the presentation, and refine the delivery. This guidance helps mentees to focus on the most relevant information and present it in a way that is both engaging and informative. After the presentation, mentors should provide specific, actionable feedback that focuses on both strengths and areas for improvement. This should be done in a supportive way that allows the mentee to reflect on their performance for further learning. Constructive feedback cannot be missed for continuous improvement in the competence and confidence of the mentee. The mentors should also encourage the mentees to plan some time to reflect on their presentation, considering what went well and what didn't, for future presentations. This reflection is a principal component in learning, whereby, after considering the remarks, the mentees can better internalize the feedback received and apply it to future presentations.

Mentees' presentations are vital component of the medical mentorship model. They provide a platform for skill development, knowledge consolidation, and professional growth. With proper guidance, preparation, and practice, mentees can excel in their presentations, gaining the confidence and competence necessary for a successful career in medicine. These experiences not only enhance their educational journey but also prepare them for the challenges they will face as medical professionals.

Long-term Impact of Presentation Skills

Having strong presentation skills in medicine does not just prove beneficial; it also propels someone through his career. Physicians who are effective in making presentations, whether in a clinical setting or in other academic contexts, become leaders in their respective disciplines. This gives a chance for teaching, research, and leadership positions that are very crucial in building a career. Communication skills, among which the presentation skill is included, are directly related to professional development and career promotion. For instance, a study evaluating the impact of faculty development programs highlighted that participants who enhanced their presentation and communication skills perceived greater success in their educator roles and had more expansive local and national networks, which are essential for career progression. Moreover, the ability to effectively communicate clinical findings or research results is often a determinant of success in securing research funding and publishing in high-impact journals. This ability, in turn, opens doors to more advanced positions within academic and clinical settings. Another study revealed that healthcare professionals who demonstrated strong presentation skills were more likely to pursue and achieve higher academic and clinical roles due to their ability to communicate complex ideas effectively and persuasively [9].

Consistently high-quality presentations establish the benchmark for a good professional reputation within the medical fraternity. The accomplished presenters are perceived as authorities over their stories, with the notion bringing them increased visibility and respect from their peers. Whereas this reputation is important for individual career growth, it is equally relevant in influencing the wider field of medicine. For instance, a long-term study on the impact of communication training among physicians found that those who had improved their presentation and communication skills were more likely to be viewed as leaders in their departments. They were also more frequently invited to speak at national and international conferences, further solidifying their professional standing. Furthermore, presentations at conferences and other professional gatherings are key opportunities for networking.

Those who can present their work get lots of valuable connections that might lead to collaborations, mentorship opportunities, and invitations to important projects. In one study concerning career impacts made via presentation skills among underrepresented minority groups, it clearly stated that those who attended programs that enhanced presentation skills did not only advance in their careers but also built considerable professional networks, which were vital in their long-term success [10].

In conclusion, the ability to deliver compelling presentations is not just about communication; it is about positioning oneself as a leader and influencer in the medical field. This skill set is a powerful tool for career advancement and for building a professional reputation that endures throughout a medical career.

Psychological Aspects and Performance Anxiety in Medical Presentations

In medicine, often regarded as a high-pressure arena, typical reactions of a mentee while preparing for and delivering a presentation would include serious psychological challenges. Left unchecked, this may impact not only the quality of the presentation but also the long-lasting confidence and professional development of the mentee.

- **Dealing with Impostor syndrome:** Impostor syndrome is a psychological phenomenon where individuals doubt their accomplishments and have a persistent fear of being exposed as a "fraud." This is particularly prevalent among medical professionals, where the stakes are high and the expectations are rigorous. Mentees may struggle with feelings of inadequacy, especially when presenting to an audience of seasoned professionals. They may believe that they don't truly belong or that their success is due to luck rather than their abilities and hard work. Research has shown that impostor syndrome is prevalent in high-achieving professions, including medicine. A study highlighted that a significant number of medical students and residents experience impostor syndrome, which can lead to increased stress, anxiety, and burnout [11]. For this reason, mentors need to thwart this by advising their mentees to concentrate on their strengths and the achievements they have made, rather than the failures or weak points thought to be found in them. Developing self-confidence may be said to be about pinpointing and celebrating these small wins and understanding how natural such mistakes may be in the learning process. An effective tool is cognitive restructuring, in which mentees learn to identify and challenge negative thoughts about what they are capable of. This approach helps to reframe their mindset, allowing them to view their achievements objectively and reduce feelings of inadequacy.

Mentors can play a critical role by providing reassurance and constructive feedback, emphasizing the mentee's progress and potential.

- **Stress management techniques:** Performance anxiety is another common issue faced by mentees during presentations. The pressure to perform well, particularly in front of an expert audience, can lead to stress, nervousness, and even physical symptoms such as sweating, shaking, or a racing heart. These symptoms can detract from the presentation and reinforce feelings of inadequacy. Effective stress management strategies are essential for helping mentees perform at their best. Some of the accepted methods include Mindfulness-Based Stress Reduction (MBSR), which incorporates deep breathing, meditation, and body scanning. Studies have proved that MBSR reduces anxiety and improves concentration, both of which are constructive in events that require maximum pressure, like presentations. Other than mindfulness, positive visualization might be a very potent tool. Encouraging mentees to visualize a successful presentation can help reduce anxiety and build confidence. This technique involves mentally rehearsing the presentation, including how they will handle potential challenges, which can make the actual experience feel more familiar and less daunting [12].

Third and last, preparation is everything. The better prepared a mentee will feel, the less likely the onset of overwhelming anxiety. This preparation includes mastery of content, as well as practicing multiple times-preferred in front of a supportive audience who can provide constructive feedback. Such practice builds familiarity and reduces the fear of the unknown. Taking the time to address the psychological aspects of presentations, such as impostor syndrome and performance anxiety, is an important part of the overall professional development that a medical mentee should have. By offering strategies for building self-confidence and managing stress, mentors support mentees in giving not only effective presentations but also building resilience in medical careers. These skills are not only relevant to the particular moment of the presentation but will be useful throughout their professional lives.

The Power of Shared Experience

One of the most rewarding aspects of mentorship is witnessing the growth and confidence of former mentees as they step into leadership roles themselves. Recently, we had the privilege of observing several of our graduates who are now accomplished professionals, return to present to a new cohort of mentees. Their session, titled *"Lessons from Our Experience,"* was more than a recounting of past events; it was a well-crafted guide on how to survive and thrive in the demanding environment of residency. They openly discussed challenges like impostor syndrome and performance anxiety, and underscored the vital role of effective communication in clinical settings.

One of the presenters spoke about overcoming performance anxiety through preparation, mindfulness, and positive visualization, strategies introduced during the mentorship. This testimony resonated deeply with the audience, offering a practical, lived example of how to navigate high-pressure scenarios with confidence. For new mentees, it was a reassuring reminder that the obstacles they now face can indeed be overcome with the right mindset and approach.

What made this peer-led presentation so impactful was its authenticity. The session revealed a core truth of our mentorship philosophy: learning doesn't only flow from top to bottom. Sometimes, the most powerful lessons come from those who have just recently walked the same path.

These returning graduates also emphasized the long-term value of mastering presentation skills, not only as a tool for communication, but as a marker of professional maturity. In teaching others, they reinforced their own knowledge and deepened their understanding. This moment captured the continuity of mentorship at its best. A cycle where former mentees evolve into mentors, keeping the spirit of the program alive.

This event reminded us all that mentorship is both a joy and a responsibility. It is about peer support, shared wisdom, and the lifelong cultivation of essential skills. By returning to guide a new generation, these graduates embodied the circular nature of mentorship. Learning from those before and lifting those who follow. It was a celebration of our community's commitment to excellence, one that continues to shape the future of medicine.

Empowering the Next Generation of Medical Researchers

Another fulfilling moment in our mentorship journey came when two of the former mentees who are now respected researchers, returned to deliver a teaching session on how to conduct effective medical research. For many of our new mentees, who were just beginning to explore the world of research, this session was more than a learning opportunity. It was a source of inspiration and clarity.

The session, titled *"A Practical Guide to Medical Research,"* offered a comprehensive, step-by-step approach to designing and executing research projects. The speakers shared the lessons they had learned throughout their own journeys, including how to frame meaningful research questions, select appropriate methodologies, and maintain rigorous scientific standards. They also emphasized the importance of aligning research with personal interest and long-term career goals. What made this session especially powerful was the way they spoke about the role of mentorship in shaping their paths. They recalled moments when the support of their mentors helped them overcome setbacks and build the confidence needed to move forward. As they passed on that wisdom to the new mentees, it was clear they were not only sharing knowledge, they were continuing the cycle of mentorship.

I could see how much this session impacted the mentees. Many were at the very beginning of their research journeys and left with a clearer sense of direction, as well as a newfound motivation. The practical advice was incredibly useful, but the personal stories were what truly moved them. They were reminded that research is not an individual endeavor but a shared mission—one that thrives on collaboration, mentorship, and persistence.

This experience reaffirmed a core belief that guides our mentorship program: when mentees are empowered, they become mentors themselves. And through that cycle, we create a lasting impact on the future of medical science.

Case Discussions and Clinical Presentations

One of the most impactful methods for deepening clinical understanding and building professional confidence in neurosurgery is through focused case discussions and clinical presentations. Recently, the mentees presented sessions on critical neurosurgical topics, showcasing not only their growing expertise but also their ability to communicate complex medical knowledge with clarity and purpose.

The presentations covered a wide range of topics, beginning with vestibular schwannoma. The speaker navigated through the diagnosis, radiological assessment, and surgical approaches, illustrating how individualized planning is central to optimal outcomes. The emphasis on recognizing clinical symptoms, such as hearing loss, tinnitus, and balance disturbance, alongside the interpretation of MRI findings, offered a structured clinical pathway for the mentees. What made the session especially effective was the nuanced discussion on surgical decision-making, which balanced risks, benefits, and patient-specific factors.

Another mentee focused on mastering brain CT interpretation. A fundamental skill in neurosurgical practice. The session walked the mentees through basic principles, from tissue density to identifying key pathologies such as hemorrhage, infarction, and tumors. Through real case studies, the mentees practiced systematic scan interpretation and were encouraged to develop consistent approaches that reduce diagnostic error.

A presentation on head trauma followed, addressing a condition that remains one of the most urgent and common challenges in neurosurgery. The discussion began with classifications of injury severity and progressed into detailed protocols for assessment, including the use of the Glasgow Coma Scale and critical imaging modalities. Updated management strategies, such as decompressive craniectomy and intracranial pressure monitoring, were explored in detail, offering the mentees insight into both emergency and post-operative care. This session effectively connected foundational knowledge with evolving surgical interventions.

We also had an enriching discussion on Moyamoya Disease, a rare but significant cerebrovascular condition. The speaker carefully explained its clinical manifestations, diagnostic strategies, and the complexity of surgical revascularization options. Discussions extended to the challenges of differentiating Moyamoya from other vasculopathies, and the importance of imaging in diagnosis and follow-up. This session reminded us that rare conditions demand not only technical knowledge, but a commitment to continued learning and research.

Another valuable session focused on brain vasculature, mapping the major arteries and veins, identifying anatomical variations, and understanding their implications in neurosurgical procedures. Vascular anomalies such as aneurysms and arteriovenous malformations were covered, along with cutting-edge treatment modalities and imaging techniques. The discussion integrated case-based problem-solving, requiring mentees to think critically about how anatomy, pathology, and decision-making intersect in real clinical practice.

What stood out in all these presentations was not only the depth of knowledge shared, but also the professionalism, clarity, and empathy with which it was communicated. Watching the mentees teach their peers, I was reminded of how powerful peer-led education can be. The mentees did not just absorb facts. They were invited to think, question, and apply. They saw examples of excellence that were both aspirational and relatable.

As I watched the mentees take the stage and share what they've learned, I saw the future of neurosurgery taking shape. And in that moment, the true meaning of mentorship became clear again: we rise by lifting others, and every lesson shared is a legacy in motion.

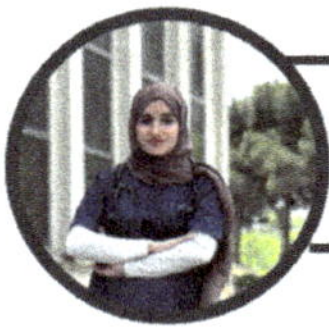

Alkawthar M. Abdulsada

A story should have a beginning, a plot, and an end, but not necessarily in the same order. To be the best in y field does not actually mean you have read every book or skimmed each paper related to the surgery you operating today. You simply have to read the right book and the right paper, and here comes the role of a men The concept of mentorship is so ubiquitous that if you think you have never seen it, you have not look Throughout history, many individuals have served as mentors, guiding and influencing others in various fields s as medicine, philosophy, science, politics, and arts.
Whether you want to be a successful general physician or a world-known hybrid vascular neurosurgeon v thousand-plus publications and letters of honour, there is only one way it should be done, and that is what the I Mentorship program taught me; The Guidelines. "We will do it the same way it is done in the United State Canada, or Germany, we will operate on our patients by the same steps written in the neurosurgical books follow international guidelines", I vividly hear Dr Hoz saying that on my first day observing the OR. Before hearing t I had been reading every medical book I encountered, trying to learn various approaches to the correct managem even though medicine is not practiced in this manner. It follows systemic methodology as the solar system ha laws and timing or as any dish is cooked following a sequential recipe, by losing international guidelines track will end up treating patients but not healing them. I learnt that walking one step in the right direction is better t a mile in the wrong non approved way.
As a first-generation medical student, the Hoz mentorship program was a treasure hunt map for me, it guided to the true path and trained me to be more serene, calm, and on purpose. It represents a universal and timeless manual particularly but not exclusively to medicine. I joined as an ordinary medical student and gained the p and confidence of a neurosurgeon. Dr Hoz has always supported me and taught me that I should give this gift a by helping other students to find their own destiny. I was in my third-year medical school when I was introdu to the program and it made a great shift in my career academically and clinically and the giving continues till to Regardless of technical challenges, there was a bigger hurdle that I was not studying in Iraq by the time I joi the team and I did not know anyone of my peers but they welcomed me as one of them and let me get familiar v their terms and many of them are now dear friends of mine. The Hoz Mentorship program taught me to be b to ask even if it is not the smartest question and to help others as long as I am able to, it always pays back in most unexpected way!

References

1. Haber RJ, Lingard LA. Learning oral presentation skills: a rhetorical analysis with pedagogical and professional implications. Journal of general internal medicine. 2001 May;16:308-14.
2. Pryor E, Ma H, Christie J. Developing clinical communication skills: targeting the postgraduate years. Medical Education. 2013 Nov 1;47(11):1141-.
3. Gibson S, Molloy E. Professional skill development needs of newly graduated health professionals: A systematic literature review. Focus on Health Professional Education: A Multi-Professional Journal. 2012 Mar 1;13(3):71-83.
4. Hammer RR, Rian JD, Gregory JK, Bostwick JM, Birk CB, Chalfant L, Scanlon PD, Hall-Flavin DK. Telling the patient's story: using theatre training to improve case presentation skills. Medical humanities. 2011 Jun 1;37(1):18-22.
5. Green EH, Hershman W, DeCherrie L, Greenwald J, Torres-Finnerty N, Wahi-Gururaj S. Developing and implementing universal guidelines for oral patient presentation skills. Teaching and learning in medicine. 2005 Jul 1;17(3):263-7.
6. Pasquale SJ, Pugnaire MP. Preparing medical students to teach. Academic Medicine. 2002 Nov 1;77(11):1175-6.
7. Clarke MA, Haggar FL, Branecki CE, Welniak TJ, Smith MP, Vasistha S, Love LM. Determining presentation skills gaps among healthcare professionals. Journal of Visual Communication in Medicine. 2022 Oct 2;45(4):242-52.
8. Watts E, Peacock O, Liyanage S, Elsey E, Lund J. Presentation skills amongst surgical trainees at a national conference: an observational study. JRSM short reports. 2012 May;3(5):1-7.
9. Morzinski J, Simposon D, Marcdante K, Meurer L, Gilligan M, Chandler T. Evaluating the career impact of faculty development using matched controls. Family medicine. 2019;51(10):841-4.
10. Gulbrandsen P, Jensen BF, Finset A, Blanch-Hartigan D. Long-term effect of communication training on the relationship between physicians' self-efficacy and performance. Patient education and counseling. 2013 May 1;91(2):180-5.

11. Clance PR, Imes SA. The imposter phenomenon in high achieving women: Dynamics and therapeutic intervention. Psychotherapy: Theory, research & practice. 1978;15(3):241.
12. Goyal M, Singh S, Sibinga EM, Gould NF, Rowland-Seymour A, Sharma R, Berger Z, Sleicher D, Maron DD, Shihab HM, Ranasinghe PD. Meditation programs for psychological stress and well-being: a systematic review and meta-analysis. JAMA internal medicine. 2014 Mar 1;174(3):357-68.
13. Hoz SS, Azeez MM, Dolachee AA, Al-Awadi OM, Moscote-Salazar LR. The new generation Iraqi neurosurgeons' armamentarium to gain the Nobel Prize, an overview of the planning and expectation for the future. Romanian Neurosurgery. 2018 Mar 15:105-9.

Section 3: Reflections and Future Directions

CH.10: Integrating National and International Experts into the Hoz Mentorship Ecosystem

The word "international collaboration" refers to a broad range of formal or informal cooperative alliances that are formed with the aim of working together to accomplish the various activities and initiatives associated with academics, such as research, education, and service/clinical practice. There seems to be an increasing trend of international collaboration in physical therapy education to improve educational programs. Collaboration on educational programs can take the form of invited lectures, international visiting professors, sharing of educational materials, sabbatical experiences, or lectures via electronic or Internet media. The development of the Internet has increased the possibilities for remote learning and collaboration in education, but it has also increased the necessity for certain adjustments. One unique aspect of international collaboration is the exchange of instructors and students across country borders. Opportunities to share exclusive data sources, postal correspondence, idea exchanges at conferences, visits to foreign labs, and paper collaboration are some aspects of international research collaboration. Formal or informal brainstorming sessions to generate research ideas, collaborative project design and execution, joint manuscript preparation and publication, and joint supervision of student research projects, including participation in thesis and dissertation committees, are some examples of the benefits of international research collaboration [1].

Healthcare professionals and leaders should approach their work with a global perspective, and internationalization can help people learn more about the significant global health education-specific concerns. Internationalization of medical education (IoME) can improve students' comprehension of social, cultural, and ethical distinctions, which will better educate aspiring doctors to practice medicine with a global perspective and a more sophisticated awareness of cultural diversity. This will eventually improve global health for everyone on the planet.

IoME can take many forms, including multiple medical education dimensions and stakeholders. It can cover subjects pertaining to teacher, curriculum, and/or student problems and experiences. Moreover, institutions, governments, or policies can all exhibit aspects of globalization [2].

The development, maintenance, and improvement of healthcare services for individuals, as well as the integrity of the healthcare system at large, are the responsibilities that society places on doctors and other healthcare professionals. Physicians must possess the necessary leadership abilities since healthcare delivery to patients and the systems supporting it continuously change over time. Medical educators need to make leadership development a regular part of their curricula in order to stay relevant. It was decided that the task of creating a medical education leadership curriculum that could be distributed and customized to local settings across the globe should be taken up by an international consortium of medical educators and other interested parties. Relational cultural theory is in favor of more extensive involvement in the advancement of healthcare leadership education. Resources used to be generated and distributed locally or regionally. Nonetheless, connection cultural theory encourages the participation of as many various contributors as possible in the co-creation of resources that are shared by all in an ever-shrinking global community. Intentionally integrating leadership development throughout the medical continuum, from undergraduate medical education to practice, promotes diversity. Reaching out to other health professionals would also enhance it. Although achieving such a comprehensive integration will require time, efforts to begin with a postgraduate curriculum shouldn't be postponed [3].

International Pioneers in Neurosurgery

In today's interconnected world, the boundaries of education and mentorship extend far beyond geographical limits. Our mentorship program has been privileged to host several international pioneers in neurosurgery who, despite the physical distances, have contributed immensely to the development of our mentees through online collaboration. These esteemed guests, each a leader in their respective fields, have brought a wealth of knowledge, cutting-edge insights, and global perspectives to our program, enriching the educational experience in ways that traditional methods alone could not achieve. Over the past year, we have been honored to welcome a series of internationally renowned neurosurgeons who have participated in our mentorship program via virtual platforms. These experts, who are at the forefront of neurosurgical innovation and research, have provided our mentees with unparalleled learning opportunities, bridging the gap between local practice and global advancements.

One such guest was Dr. Federico Nicolosi from Italy, a pioneer in minimally invasive neurosurgery. Renowned for his endoscopic skull base surgery, Dr. Nicolosi shared years of experience with our mentees through a live virtual workshop. Direct interaction with Dr. Nicolosi himself, asking questions, and receiving the entire experience came out to be invaluable for them in augmenting their understanding and skills manifold.

Another distinguished guest was Dr. Silky Chotai from the United States, a leading expert in cerebrovascular neurosurgery. Dr. Chotai is renowned for her pioneering techniques in the treatment of complex aneurysms and arteriovenous malformations (AVMs). This collaboration not only broadened their clinical knowledge but also inspired them to think creatively and push the boundaries of conventional treatment methods.

Dr. Woralux Phusoongnern of Thailand is an internationally recognized expert in pediatric neurosurgery and has also joined our mentorship program through online collaboration. Dr. Phusoongnern is globally renowned for her contribution to the development of novel surgical techniques in treating congenital brain disorders. After participating in our mentorship program, Dr. Phusoongnern underlined that special training and continuous education are necessary to satisfy the ever-evolving neurosurgical needs.

We were also honored to host Dr. Baha'Eddin Muhsen from Jordan and practice US, an expert in spinal neurosurgery. Dr. Muhsen's contributions to advancing techniques in minimally invasive spinal surgery have made significant impacts on patient outcomes worldwide. Dr. Muhsen's hands-on approach to virtual teaching allowed mentees to engage with real surgical cases, enhancing their practical understanding and decision-making skills. Thereafter, Dr. Giath Al-Dayri in Germany took over with his specialty neurosurgery. His work has pioneered new techniques in developing new approaches to the surgical management of brain tumors. Advanced technology that can help improve patient outcomes in difficult cases where the conventional approach is not feasible decidedly drew the interests of the mentees.

In addition to these renowned figures, our program was further enriched by contributions from Dr. QADAMXER R. HAMA, Dr. Elena Nestian, and Dr. Margreda Concecao. Their impact on our program was profound. Each brought unique expertise and perspectives that resonated deeply with our mentees.

This participation of the international pioneers in our mentorship greatly inspires and influences the mentality of our mentees. Similarly, interaction with such global leaders opens our mentees to state-of-the-art concepts in neurosurgery, many of which have not diffused into the general medical scene. This inspired our mentees to pursue excellence in their careers and contribute to forward movement in the field by affording them a unique opportunity for direct learning from those shaping the future of neurosurgery.

These online collaborations have also demonstrated the power of technology in overcoming the limitations of distance, enabling our program to provide a truly global educational experience. The interactions with these experts have not only enhanced the technical skills of our mentees but have also broadened their understanding of how neurosurgery is practiced in different cultural and healthcare contexts. This global perspective is invaluable, as it prepares our mentees to be more adaptable and innovative in their future practices. By connecting our mentees with pioneers in neurosurgery from around the world, we have not only expanded their knowledge and skills but also fostered a global network of mentorship and collaboration. This network will continue to grow and evolve, ensuring that our mentees are equipped with the knowledge, confidence, and inspiration to lead in the ever-advancing field of neurosurgery.

Principles for Successful International Collaborations

Over the years, through our personal experiences and numerous conversations with colleagues around the world, we have synthesized several key principles that are essential for the successful development of international collaborations and projects in the field of neurosurgery. These principles have been instrumental in guiding our efforts to build robust, productive, and sustainable partnerships that advance both medical education and clinical practice.

- **Shared vision and goals:** One of the cornerstones of any successful international collaboration is a developed and shared vision and mission. In our collective experience, the most productive collaborations arise when there is clarity of alignment regarding goals by all parties concerned. Whether it be research, clinical outcomes, or medical education, the better defined and mutually agreed the purpose, the greater the chances of success in partnership. In our collaboration with institutions abroad, we have found that this has to do with early discussions to articulate shared goals. That clarity helps to ensure that all partners are working toward the same outcomes, reducing misunderstandings and misaligned expectations downstream in the project.

- **Cultural sensitivity and mutual respect:** International collaborations bring together individuals from diverse cultural backgrounds, each with their own practices, values, and expectations. From our interactions with global colleagues, we've learned that cultural sensitivity and mutual respect are critical to building trust and fostering effective communication. Understanding and appreciating cultural differences has allowed us to navigate potential challenges more effectively and to create an inclusive environment where all participants feel valued and respected. This cultural awareness not only strengthens the collaboration but also enriches the learning experience for everyone involved.
- **Open and transparent communication:** Smooth communication is the lifeblood of successful collaboration. We have learned through experience that open and transparent lines of communication throughout a project's life provide the necessary foundation for success. Regular updates, transparent record-keeping, and frank discussions of challenges and expectations are some of the basic tenets of building trust and engaging all partners. We found this to be particularly effective in using technology through video conferencing and collaborative platforms to help bridge the gap in communications across different time zones and distances. The benefit of these types of tools is that we could have one single, ongoing dialogue with international partners that keeps everyone on the same page.
- **Flexibility and adaptability:** International collaborations often involve navigating different healthcare systems, regulatory environments, and resource constraints. From our work on various global projects, we've learned that flexibility and adaptability are key to overcoming these challenges. Being open to adjusting timelines, modifying objectives, or exploring alternative approaches has allowed us to keep projects on track, even when faced with unforeseen obstacles. This adaptability not only helps to ensure the success of the project but also demonstrates a commitment to the partnership, fostering a sense of mutual support and collaboration.
- **Long-term commitment and sustainability:** Successful international collaboration is a long-term commitment by the parties concerned. In our experience, we have noticed that sustainable partnerships are only possible if their foundation is continuous interaction and learning. We have managed to establish long-term relationships with international partners by investing in the development of long-lasting projects. This involves planning the

sustainability of the collaboration beyond the actual period of the project through continuous training, initiation of research work, or building capacity. As it were, in focusing on sustainability, we ensure that the impacts of the collaboration will still be felt long after the close of the project.

- **Mutual benefit and reciprocity:** For an international collaboration to be truly successful, it must be mutually beneficial. Through our projects, we have prioritized ensuring that all partners gain value from the collaboration, whether it's through access to new knowledge, resources, or opportunities for professional growth. We've found that when all parties feel that they are contributing to and benefiting from the collaboration, the partnership is more likely to be strong and enduring. This sense of reciprocity not only strengthens the bond between collaborators but also enhances the overall impact of the project.
- **Leveraging networks and building capacity:** We have learned the value of tapping into existing networks and concentrating on capacity building in international partnerships. The art of networking through already established networks and engaging key stakeholders has helped us expand our projects both in outreach and impact. Indeed, the approach toward local capacity building has been one of the key factors in our international work. We seek to enhance the capacity of our international partners through various training programs, workshops, and joint research activities so that the outcome of this collaboration will be sustainable and have a wider reach.

Our experiences and conversations with colleagues worldwide have provided us with valuable insights into the principles that underpin successful international collaborations. By focusing on shared goals, cultural sensitivity, clear communication, flexibility, long-term commitment, mutual benefit, and capacity building, we have been able to develop partnerships that are not only productive but also enduring. These principles have guided our efforts to create meaningful and impactful collaborations that advance the field of neurosurgery and enhance medical education on a global scale.

Obstacles in Global Scientific Cooperation

All parties involved benefit when people from diverse cultural backgrounds collaborate with one another. These alliances, nonetheless, may also present unanticipated difficulties. Involving people from other cultures and countries in initiatives can be beneficial for the advancement of science.

But it also comes with unique challenges, possible risks, and disadvantages. Here are some of the key challenges faced in international collaborations:

1. **Language barriers:** Language differences can lead to misunderstandings, misinterpretation of instructions, and reduced effectiveness in communication. This can impact everything from daily interactions to the interpretation of complex medical or research data. Even when collaborators speak the same language, differences in medical terminology and professional jargon across regions can cause confusion.
2. **Cultural differences:** It is crucial to keep in mind that cultural differences affect the way members from different cultures communicate, make decisions, and behave at work. What is considered appropriate, polite, or proper in one culture may not be seen the same in another culture. Different standards and/or practices of host country ethics Quite often create conflict on how research should be carried out.
3. **Time zone differences:** Working across multiple time zones can make scheduling meetings and coordinating project timelines difficult. The lack of overlap in working hours often leads to delays in communication and decision-making. Teams may have to rely heavily on asynchronous communication (e.g., emails and recorded meetings), which can slow down the pace of collaboration and create bottlenecks in project progress.
4. **Funding and resource allocation:** Disparities in funding and resources between collaborating institutions can create power imbalances. Institutions with more resources may have more influence over the direction and priorities of the collaboration, which can lead to tensions. Securing long-term funding for international projects can be challenging. Differences in funding cycles, priorities of funding bodies, and economic conditions in different countries can affect the continuity of the collaboration.
5. **Logistical and operational challenges:** The collaborators may have problems with visa issues, restrictions in traveling, and lack of funds for travel that would create barriers to face-to-face communications, which are often the benchmarks upon which a trusting, understanding relationship is founded. Besides that, infrastructural differences in internet connectivity, laboratory facilities, and technological access bring in a number of challenges for ensuring that such collaboration is provided on equal grounds.

Addressing these challenges requires careful planning, clear communication, cultural sensitivity, and a commitment to finding solutions that work for all parties involved. By acknowledging and proactively managing these challenges, international collaborations can achieve their full potential, leading to meaningful and impactful outcomes.

Dandy Pan Arab Meeting 2022 Experience

A neurosurgery conference was held at the American University of Beirut (AUB) in 2022 by the Walter E. Dandy Neurosurgery Club; its main audience was neurosurgeons and individuals with a general interest in neurosurgery, which also included medical students and residents. The conference consisted of two days, and the schedule included multiple speakers, most of them were neurosurgeons presenting a part of their experience or a snapshot of their specialty.

Dr. Samer Hoz was one of the main speakers invited to this conference. What made this experience distinctive and related to the mentorship essence is that many of the students who attended the conference were his mentees during one of the mentorship cycles, and the most unique thing was that it wasn't planned, yet a team of 10 students made it to the conference coincidentally with their mentor, providing him and each other with support and confidence.

Three of those mentees were also speakers at this conference, and they presented 3 abstracts from projects they have contributed to. Eventually, two of them placed within the top 5 best abstracts and were awarded for it. It was very clear how knowledgeable and interested they were in what they were presenting; this stems from the fact that these weren't just research projects they had a part in, in fact, it was mostly the stories of how they got the opportunity that made them motivated enough to put much effort and work in everything they participated in.

On the other hand, the mentor, Dr. Samer Hoz, gave one of the most influential presentations at the conference with the title of "Bridging the gap between medical students and neurosurgeons." The presentation consisted of two main segments. The first segment included several unique cases he had encountered, presented in a step-by-step approach with a volunteer from the crowd answering the questions related to the anatomy observed and the case itself; it was an intriguing form of presentation as it didn't only show the clinical aspect of the case. Moreover, it showed glimpses of how neurosurgery improves patients' lives, this part of the presentation also introduced some of the team's publications based on unique cases and experiences. The second segment introduced the concept of the Hoz neurosurgery mentorship; this segment was portrayed by selected mentees' stories. Each story highlighted the experience each mentee gained from the beginning of the mentorship until that very moment; this varied from clinical experience, OR attendance, endovascular knowledge and assistance, and research experience; at the end of each story, the student is asked to stand up so the audience can see them. This initiative had multiple positive impacts on both the general audience and the mentees themselves. Relaying experiences in story form can motivate people to pursue their goals and learn more. Additionally, it gives the mentioned individual, the mentee, a considerable amount of confidence and a feeling of achievement, as there is no greater encouragement than the acknowledgment of efforts and hard work, especially by loved ones in the audience and people with similar interests.

This conference facilitated various opportunities for networking between students and neurosurgeons. There was a common feeling of understanding and validation felt even by the youngest medical students. The statement of being present as a team during the conference, along with this essential presentation, highlighted the key features of this mentorship. Therefore, a generally positive impression was made, many people had questions about how they could join the mentorship or have a parallel experience from a different region of the world and with their mentors. Many new mentees were now part of the Hoz mentorship and were even included in research teams and projects that came later.

This gathering has provided an opportunity for the mentees to reflect on their past experiences and address their future goals. After each day of the conference, the team would meet to have collective feedback and shed light on the most influential and inspiring moments of this experience. This opportunity was also a chance to reminisce about the motivation that drives people toward excellence and how a person is far more successful if he is on a team or being guided in the right direction by the right person. The importance of having a mentor in one's life, especially medical students, became distinctively clear during those few days.

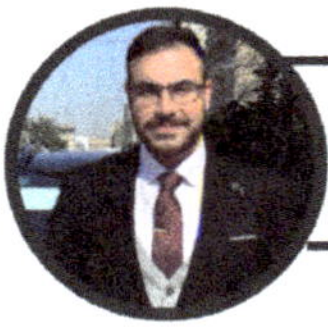

Mustapha Murayati

Neurosurgery mentorship has been one of the most transformative experiences in my professional journey. It sta as I was a fresh medical student in early medical school years who is fascinated about the complexity and challer in neurosciences. At first putting all brain part together was challenging. As a mentee, I've realized that true gro begins from the willingness to be persevering, ambition, and actively seek feedback, especially the negative c that as I believe, build stronger resilience for facing future challenges.

Many valuable lessons have been learned, one of which is the importance of being part of a team. It's not just a acquiring scientific knowledge but developing a sense of trust and mutual respect that allows for open dialo and constructive criticism. As I have been in that mentorship team, it felt like a mixture of family, friend professional relationship all together in one nurturing environment. I was taught what a real teamwork looks and how to build one. My mentor taught me how to navigate personal, ethical and professional challenges, grace and confidence.

The mentorship experience also highlighted the power of collaboration. By being in a supportive environment engaging with diverse perspectives, I gained a broader understanding of the field and learned to appro challenges with a more practical view. My mentor encouraged me to think beyond borders, both literally figuratively, and this broadened my ambitions to work on a global scale. It wasn't just about indivi achievements but about contributing to a larger team and pushing boundaries together.

In reflecting on my journey, I am deeply grateful for the opportunities to connect with supportive mentors peers. These interactions have not only expanded my knowledge but also strengthened my commitmen mentorship, recognizing the responsibility to pass on what I've learned. I hope to inspire others just as I have b inspired, and I look forward to continuing this journey of learning, growth, and collaboration.

One of the key takeaways was learning to embrace failure as an opportunity for growth, which shifted perspective on setbacks and helped me develop resilience by gaining new skills. Finaly, I belive that mentorsh just like the seeds you implanted and provide it with basic nutrition and after a while you find it already grov into a fruitful tree of achievements.

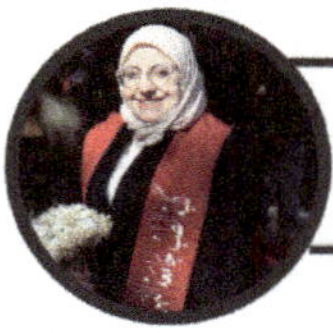

Zainab K. A. Alaraji

Iy journey with Dr. Hoz's mentorship has been nothing short of transformative.
s a first-generation medical student, my path was initially filled with uncertainty, navigating the complexities of edicine without guidance. That changed when I attended a neurosurgery conference in Beirut, Lebanon, where I nexpectedly encountered Dr. Hoz and his team. From the very first interaction, he welcomed us warmly, inviting s to join the team dinner.

was captivated by the depth of wisdom in his words, the ethical discussions, and the invaluable lessons shared. s his team spoke about their experiences, I was amazed at the immense opportunities he provided—ranging from rly clinical exposures to high-level scientific research. It was shocking to realize that medical students could be volved in such advanced projects so early in their careers. However, what truly resonated with me was the ofound guidance and mentorship he offered, not just in medicine but in life as well. A few months later, in my urth year of medical school, I joined my first research project during the mentorship. Research had always trigued me, particularly identifying gaps in the literature, and under Dr. Hoz's guidance, that passion flourished.

eyond research, his mentorship opened doors to invaluable experiences, allowing me to meet and learn from stinguished professors and surgeons—each with immense knowledge and wisdom shaped by years of experience. heir insights enriched my understanding of neurosurgery and neuroscience, offering perspectives that extended eyond textbooks. Meeting Dr. Hoz in Lebanon marked the beginning of an incredible journey—one filled with allenges but also unwavering support. Now, in my final year of medical school, with five publications and five going projects, I have gained not only a deep understanding of my field but also lessons in resilience, critical inking, and personal growth. Looking back, what initially appeared to be a coincidence, Dr. Hoz often says, is ear proof that "everything happens for a reason—there are no coincidences in life."

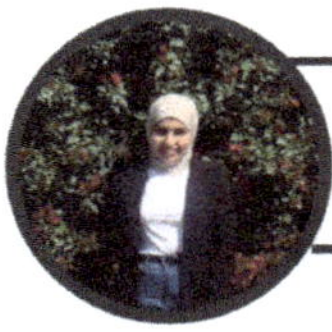

Zahraa A. Alsubaihawi

I am a newly graduated medical doctor interested in neurosurgery as a future career. In my early years of medi
school, I always thought of neurosurgeons as role models facing the most interesting part of our body, our bra
and neurosurgery as an unreachable branch that is difficult, competitive, and requires a lot of training years.
During my second year, specifically during summer vacation, I found a mentorship program added to most medi
and surgical specialties introduced by one of the medical students' associations in Iraq. Without thought, I cho
the neurosurgery mentorship program by Dr. Samer S. Hoz, and this was the beginning of my journey.
At that time, I was very shy and had no confidence in dealing with such a difficult branch, but it was interestir
The mentorship program introduced by Dr. Hoz includes teaching neurological examination, lectures about t
most common neurosurgical cases we can face, attending outpatient clinics, neurosurgery emergency departme
and surgeries. It was a simulation of how neurosurgery residents live their lives.
working on every participant's weak point, he believed in my potential when I was not. during the mentorsh
period, I decided to take every single opportunity he offered me as a challenge which resulted in presenting tw
seminars regarding neurosurgical anatomy, meningioma types, and started working to improve my academ
writing. Even after the mentorship period, he did not hesitate to help anyone.
When I first joined the mentorship, I did not have any publications or anything to build up my CV, now af
graduation, I have more than twenty published papers in international journals, participated in multiple conferenc
workshops, and book publications, have a more wide, clear vision of how my future could be. I did not imagi
that I could reach such things in my life. As a young medical student trying to find his capabilities and having ve
limited awareness about future opportunities, Dr. Hoz was the perfect role model and mentor for us. I will alwa
be grateful to him; I always tell Dr. Hoz that there are no enough words to thank him. I hope that we as a team w
achieve something in the future that will make his effort worth it.

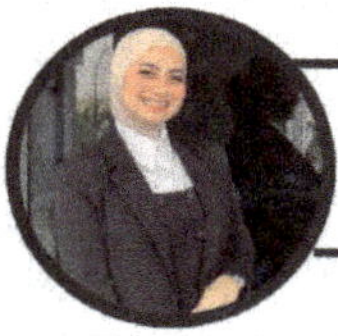

Hagar A. Algburi

othing significant in your journey than someone influence you to step out of your comfort zone.
. my 2nd year as a medical student, I had my interest in neuroscience, but I didn't know how to shape this passion how to start with. In the same year I found Hoz mentorship program that I was not so familiar with the impact such mentorship on my personality and future.

started as an eager student to learn from every meeting with such an inspiring and role model, staring with the rst task from Dr Hoz to draw a sketch for one of his papers, the proud feelings for the 1st paper included your ıme was incredible as you are just a 2nd year student. Followed by the first neurosurgery attendance, first book ıared with your fine touches and first international meeting for you.

'ith my 20 publications now, I still remember that passing these milestones as they're being in the start, it was ıpossible without supportive mentor guide the pathway based on your plans and dreams.
ıe biggest perspective I've learned from the mentorship projects that there's no limit for your capability, and for 'ery big achievement you are enough to do more than this. Dr Hoz faith in his team made them put their selves any stressful tasks by knowing that they will achieve this at the end.

om the other side, we all in Hoz mentorship faced some setbacks and failure but he taught us that mistakes are ecessary parts of our successful journey and that every mistake is an opportunity for a next level.
eamwork was the fundamental part of Dr Hoz mentoring focused on collaboration and complement each other's rength in a challenge projects. This create supportive environment where big achievements were done, and ccess were shared.

eeting Dr. Hoz for me not only meeting some one that guide your academic passion but one that shaping me into ore confident and resilient person, and as I will soon start my postgraduate life, I will try my best to carry every sson I've learned from, staring from Dr. Hoz quote;
)ur duty in life is to support each other and make the next generation even better".

References

1. Fell DW, Kim K. Developing international collaborations in physical therapy academia: a case example emphasizing education and scholarship. Journal of Physical Therapy Education. 2012 Jan 1;26(1):6-12.
2. Wu A, Noël GP, Wingate R, Kielstein H, Sakurai T, Viranta-Kovanen S, Chien CL, Traxler H, Waschke J, Vielmuth F, Sagoo MG. An international partnership of 12 anatomy departments–improving global health through internationalization of medical education. Annals of global health. 2020;86(1).
3. Chan MK, de Camps Meschino D, Dath D, Busari J, Bohnen JD, Samson LM, Matlow A, Sánchez-Mendiola M. Collaborating internationally on physician leadership development: why now?. Leadership in Health Services. 2016 Jul 4;29(3):231-9.

Section 3: Reflections and Future Directions

CH.11: Capturing Mentee Perspectives through Testimonials and Reflections

As we reach the end of this book, the heart of any mentorship program is the mentees themselves. Throughout their journey, the mentees have not only gained knowledge and skills but have shaped their identities as medical professionals. Their perspectives and feedback are invaluable in perceiving insights on the effectiveness of the program, thus giving a clear view of its strengths and areas that need improvement. The reflections in this chapter will deepen by giving a voice to our mentees concerning experiences and the impact of mentorship received.

For many mentees, this mentorship program has indeed been a transformative experience from uncertainty to confidence. The following reflections indicate how the program shaped their personal and professional growth.

- **Clinical confidence**: "When I first started, I was hesitant and unsure of my abilities. The mentorship program provided me with the guidance and support I needed to develop my clinical skills and build confidence in my decision-making. The hands-on experience and constructive feedback from my mentors were invaluable." – *Student. A,*
- **Communication skills**: " I think one of the deepest changes that I have felt within myself has to do with the way that I speak. I used to be absolutely terrified of any manner of presentation. Through consistently being faced with practice and mentorship, I have learned how to take very complex information and present it in a very clear and confident manner. This not only helps me improve my presentations but also greatly enhances my interactions with patients and colleagues." – *Student. B,*
- **Research acumen**: "The focus on research in our program has been a game-changer for me. I've learned how to conduct meaningful research, from designing a study to publishing my findings. This experience has ignited a passion for academic medicine that I didn't know I had." – *Student C,*
- **Global Perspective**: "Participating in sessions with international experts like Dr. Federico Nicolosi and Dr. Silky Chotai was incredibly inspiring. It was fascinating to learn about

the different approaches to neurosurgery in other countries and how these can be applied in our own practice. These collaborations have given me a more global perspective on medicine." – *Student. D,*

Areas for Improvement

While the general feedback has been positive, there have also been constructive comments by mentees, which point to areas where the program might need improvement. This is important for the continued development of the Mentorship Program:

- **More personalized mentorship**: "The program is excellent, but I think it could benefit from more personalized mentorship. Sometimes, the group sessions don't address the specific challenges I'm facing in my specialty. More one-on-one time with mentors could help address these individual needs." – *Student E,*
- **Expanded research opportunities**: " This has really been great research training; what I want to see more about, however, is opportunities in collaborating on international research projects. This will give us much more experience regarding research, but also a valuable contribution to the advancement of health globally." – *Student F,*
- **Integration of wellness support**: "The program is intense, and while the mentorship is great, I think we could benefit from more support around wellness and managing stress. Burnout is a real concern, and having more resources in this area would be really valuable." – *Student G,*

Identified Challenges and Areas for Improvement

One of the primary concerns raised by mentees is that group mentorship sessions, while valuable, often fail to address individual needs, particularly those related to specific specialties. This challenge is further amplified by the sheer number of mentees participating in the program, making it impractical for a single mentor to dedicate one-on-one time to every mentee consistently. While the traditional mentorship model relies on mentees proactively seeking opportunities and demonstrating initiative, the rapid expansion of the program necessitates a more structured approach. With an increasingly global pool of mentees, ranging from beginners to advanced participants, it is essential to implement a system that ensures every mentee receives guidance tailored to their stage of development. To address this challenge, we propose a tiered mentorship system that enhances personalization while maintaining efficiency. This structured approach consists of three core components:

1. **Establishing a Clear Pathway for Mentee Growth:** A well-defined roadmap outlining the journey from novice to advanced levels is crucial for ensuring that mentees can track their progress and understand the expectations at each stage. This roadmap should include a set of core competencies and skills required at each level, guidelines for success, including milestones that mentees must achieve to progress, and leadership development pathways, ensuring that mentees evolve into future mentors and contributors.
2. **Implementing a Multi-Level Mentee Structure:** To create a more organized and scalable system, mentees will be divided into different levels based on experience and progress. These levels include Junior Mentees, who are entry-level participants still exploring foundational skills and knowledge; Intermediate Mentees, who have gained experience and are actively contributing to discussions, research, or clinical activities; and Senior Mentees, who are experienced individuals taking on leadership roles in guiding junior and intermediate mentees. Each senior mentee will be responsible for mentoring a small group of junior or intermediate mentees, ensuring that guidance is distributed effectively. This system fosters peer-to-peer learning while reducing the burden on primary mentors.
3. **Leveraging a Digital Dashboard for Mentee Progress Tracking:** To facilitate structured mentorship, we propose using Notion (or a similar platform) as a centralized hub where mentees can document their progress through structured milestones, receive feedback from senior mentees and mentors, and track their participation in research, discussions, and clinical case studies. Senior mentees will play a crucial role in maintaining and updating these progress boards, ensuring that mentors have quick access to summary reports rather than manually reviewing each mentee's work.

A Systematic Approach to Address Direct Mentor-Mentee Interaction

While one-on-one mentorship remains a cornerstone of effective training, it is logistically unfeasible for a single mentor to engage directly with a large cohort of over 100 mentees. To preserve the quality of mentor-mentee interactions while ensuring accessibility and personalization, we propose a structured, scalable approach.

First, a Structured Request System will be implemented to streamline direct mentor engagement. Mentees seeking individualized guidance must submit a formal request through their assigned senior mentee. Each submission should include a concise summary of the mentee's progress within the program, a well-defined query or topic necessitating discussion, and a clear justification for the need for a one-on-one meeting. This process not only fosters intentionality in communication but also ensures that mentor interactions are meaningful and focused on areas of genuine need. Furthermore, it cultivates the mentee's ability to articulate concerns and prioritize objectives—essential skills in both academic and clinical settings. To complement this, mentors will establish Designated Consultation Slots to replace ad hoc meetings. These scheduled sessions will be allocated based on the urgency and relevance of the submitted requests, ensuring that the mentor's time is used efficiently while maximizing the value of each interaction.

An observed barrier to creativity within mentorship programs is the reluctance of mentees to share ideas due to self-doubt or fear of criticism. To address this, the integration of an Ideas & Innovation Section within the mentorship framework is proposed. This initiative will encourage mentees to document and present innovative concepts related to research, clinical practice, or the structure of the mentorship program itself. Structured guidelines will be provided to help mentees effectively articulate their proposals, and intellectual ownership of contributions will be maintained.

Senior mentees and designated coordinators will serve as the initial reviewers of these proposals, offering constructive feedback and refinement prior to presentation to primary mentors. This process fosters a culture of creativity, reduces psychological barriers, and empowers mentees to actively participate in the evolution of the program.

The intensity of structured mentorship programs, while beneficial, can inadvertently contribute to stress and burnout among mentees. To proactively address these challenges, a Wellness and Support Component will be embedded within the framework. A dedicated Concerns & Challenges Section will allow mentees to confidentially express issues related to workload, emotional stress, or academic pressure. These inputs will be analyzed and synthesized into Monthly Wellness

Reports, which highlight common themes and enable mentors to take targeted action to alleviate systemic stressors.

Moreover, mentees will be encouraged to engage in daily self-reflection and mindfulness exercises. Structured guidance will be provided on how to document these reflections, promoting self-awareness and resilience. This holistic approach aims to cultivate a psychologically supportive environment conducive to both personal and professional development.

The proposed multi-level, modular mentorship structure represents a transformative step toward a more efficient, inclusive, and sustainable mentorship model. By incorporating technological tools, defined progression pathways, and clearly delineated roles, the system balances individualized attention with scalability. It empowers senior mentees, optimizes the mentor's time, and enables each participant to contribute meaningfully to the collective growth of the program.

This strategic evolution is not merely a refinement of current practices; it is a forward-looking initiative designed to amplify the impact of mentorship tenfold. It ensures that mentees are not only recipients of knowledge but also active contributors to the program's ongoing development. By embedding leadership training, innovation, and wellness into the core structure, the model lays the foundation for the emergence of a resilient, skilled, and visionary generation of professionals. As Henry Ford aptly stated, "If you always do what you've always done, you'll always get what you've always got." Embracing this evolution is not only necessary—it is imperative for elevating the mentorship experience and realizing the full potential of every mentee involved.

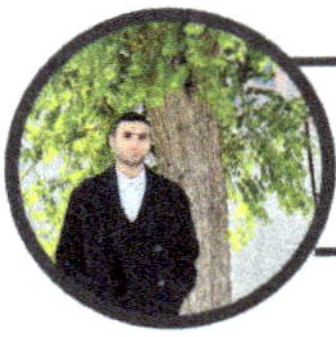

Mohammed S. Al-Baldawi

The moment when the world changed—did it really change? When, how, and why?

For me, that moment was real. It happened the day I discovered my mentor and the incredible mentorship program I've been to join. That discovery didn't just alter how I saw my future—it reshaped how I saw the world itself.

Before we dive deeper, there's something important to consider. We often assume that because we all live in the same wo experience it similarly. But that's simply not true. Each of us carries a unique version of the world in our mind—shaped perceptions, experiences, and the people who influence us. Let's think about it practically. Imagine two different people: o spends most of their day playing video games, and another who spends time reading, socializing, and gathering experiences. their descriptions of their worlds match? Absolutely not. That illustrates the point perfectly—the world continuously shifts f of us, depending on how we live, what we experience, and how our brains interpret everything around us. Speaking of the bra remarkable structure has always fascinated me. Its complexity and power to shape perception are precisely what sparked m interest in neuroscience and ultimately led me to this mentorship.

I'm Mohammed Safaa, a fifth-year medical student. My journey with the Hoz Neurosurgery Mentorship Program began dur second year of medical school. A friend introduced me after hearing how passionate I was about the brain. What astonished that everything in this mentorship—meetings, surgeries, even meals—was completely free. The only requirement was genuine and a willingness to learn. It felt too good to be true, but it was exactly what I needed, Alhamdulillah.

Initially, I joined as a curious student balancing medical school responsibilities with something I deeply loved. I couldn't fully immediately. But a few months later, I decided to revisit the group's older messages to catch up on anything I'd missed—I hac in December 2021, seven months after the mentorship officially started in May. That's when I found a voice message from I that truly shifted my perspective. In it, he emphasized that the only requirement to benefit from the mentorship was passi sincere interest. Those words resonated deeply within me. That was the exact moment my world genuinely began to change.

Unlike many mentees, my first interaction with the mentorship wasn't through an online meeting or a welcome session—it person, directly in the operating room. That experience created a unique bond between me and the heart of the program. I remember that day—February 26, 2022. It marked the first time I participated in a neurosurgical operation, helping in sn meaningful ways. It offered a brief view into the world I had always dreamed of, leaving a lasting and profound impact. Dur day, the values I deeply admired—honesty, teamwork, responsibility—came to life before my eyes. After the surgery, I unforgettable conversation with Dr. Hoz. I still remember clearly how I told him, "I want to think exactly like you," words si coming from my heart, reflecting my deep admiration and desire to adopt his approach to thinking. In that same conversation, Dr. Hoz about the USMLE Steps, and he promptly guided me to Mustafa Ismail, who had recently passed his exams at th Back then, I was just a second-year medical student, far from even thinking I could achieve such a milestone myself.

Thanks to Allah, through this mentorship, I gained the confidence I needed to start my own USMLE journey. Eventual confidence carried me through, and Alhamdulillah, I successfully passed the USMLE Step 1. This achievement wasn't jus passing an exam—it was about realizing how mentorship could unlock potential I didn't even realize I had. That unfor conversation, along with everything I experienced in the mentorship program, motivated me to take my journey seriously. my mentorship—but my life. I began to participate more actively, learn more deeply, and grow in ways I hadn't expected. I me that this journey isn't merely about acquiring knowledge—it's about becoming someone who shares and supports other the way.

The mentorship gave me opportunities beyond my imagination. More importantly, it showed me the true meaning of comm purposeful growth, continuous learning—and leadership. For all this, I'm deeply grateful—to my mentor, this mentorship, path that taught me one of life's most powerful lessons:

You should never walk alone.

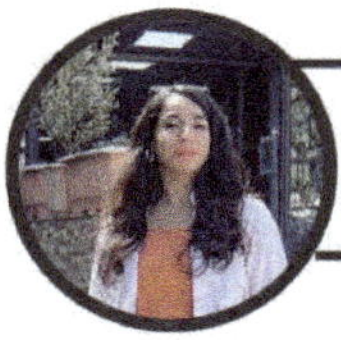

Sura Hamid

I entered my clinical years in college, I found myself searching for a deeper sense of purpose, I was looking for ɔortunities to develop beyond the scheduled routine of coursework and exams, that's when I joined the HOZ ırosurgery mentorship. I remember vividly the first meeting with Dr. Hoz when he asked us to search our name ȝoogle to be revised by the end of the program. Unsurprisingly, the results yielded nothing, that was the testament the growth and contributions we had along the way.

e first time I got into the operating room, the first research paper I authored and the first presentation I delivered ·ing the mentorship, these are milestones I will cherish throughout my career. I believe that early exposure to ıctical experience and hands-on training has shaped me both professionally and personally. It helped me develop leeper understanding of my interests, strength and potential paths and ultimately fostered my confidence to ɔome a decision maker.

e of the most valued lessons I learned is the importance of teamwork, that if we rise, we rise together. As I had ·viously navigated an environment that's highly competitive, that principle was eye-opening to me. I came to ɔreciate that progress is most meaningful when it's achieved as a team, a principle that I will always hold dear.

the end of the mentorship, I became a more confident, disciplined and enthusiastic than I have ever been. The ɔerience has not only given me opportunities but also taught me the mindset to create them. This transformation ended beyond academics, I learned that to be successful is about actively shaping my own path.

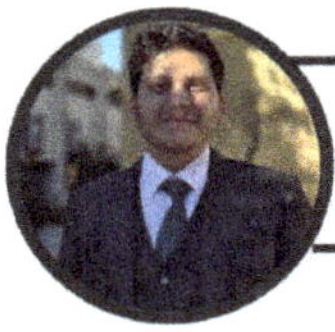

Ibrahim A. Farooq

The person who chases two rabbits catches neither. We are forever indebted to those who carried us. Havin mentor was crucial in shaping my personal and professional growth as I pursued the very reason I went to med school for Neurosurgery. This mentorship helped me focus on what truly mattered rather than getting overwhelr by distractions. Through it I understood the difficulty of accomplishing great things in isolation… Teamw collaborations, and learning from others are essential in such a demanding field, reinforcing a crucial life less greed serves no purpose, neither in neurosurgery nor life. True success is not the personal gain, but the dedicat selflessness, and the impact one leaves behind.

My name appeared in few papers and books throughout this mentorship, yet the satisfaction they brought incomparable to the joy of completing a project that has been sent back for editing multiple times. After all an e remains unseen until another's keen eye calls it forth. It helped me attend surgeries, and the discussions it brou before, after, and through the surgeries, understanding the field's precision and the relentless progress it dema only to deepen my passion for this field.

I was introduced to this mentorship in my late fourth year facing a challenging start. A poorly timed joke led to rejection, but persistence earned me a place. I began by observing others, gradually working my way to leadi team project, the experience was enriched by attending seminars from worldwide doctors sharing their insights answering our questions, as a wise doctor once said, "No question is ever stupid"

I would encourage anyone to join this program. It is an opportunity not just to gain knowledge and skills bu form connections that will support and inspire you throughout your career.

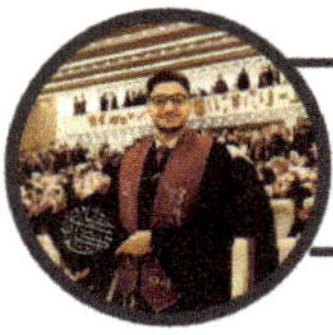

Bandar M. Al-Hadeethi

t the beginning of my medical journey, I was searching for direction, a structured path to understand different ranches of medicine, identify where my passion lay, and most importantly, figure out how to start my research ourney. I knew research was a crucial part of academic and professional growth, yet I lacked clear guidance on here to begin. I felt there was a gap between my ambition and the available resources, and I needed a system that ould provide structured learning and mentorship to help me navigate this path.

hat turning point came when I discovered the Hoz Neurosurgery Mentorship Program. I learned about it through osts from students who had been part of the program the previous year, sharing their transformative experiences. heir insights induced me to contact Dr Hoz and apply. Once I joined, I was introduced to a world of structured entorship, where I gained hands-on exposure to research, access to neurosurgical discussions, and a community at fostered both learning and collaboration.

ne of the most defining aspects of my mentorship experience has been my research development. Before joining, had no published work and lacked a clear understanding of how research projects progressed from conception to ompletion. Through the guidance of Dr. Samer Hoz and my colleagues, I gained firsthand experience in the entire esearch process from idea generation to data collection, analysis, and final publication. Attending research-focused oom sessions further deepened the understanding. This exposure transformed research from an intimidating oncept into an essential part of my academic growth. Through the mentorship I had my first publication and I am ctively working on multiple projects, applying the knowledge and experience gained through this mentorship.

longside research, the mentorship provided me with valuable exposure to neurosurgical education. I participated neuroanatomy sessions, surgical observations, and case-based discussions, allowing me to gain deeper insights to the attitude among the specialists themselves, with the other colleagues and with the family beside witnessing omplex neurosurgical procedures. Attending multidisciplinary team (MDT) meetings with senior neurosurgeons ave me firsthand experience of how critical decisions are made in real-world settings. These experiences have rengthened my understanding of neurosurgery and its challenges.

hat makes this mentorship truly unique is its self-sustaining cycle. Just as I learned from those who joined before e, I now find myself guiding newer members, helping them navigate the same challenges I once faced. Each entee is both a learner and a teacher, creating a continuous loop of knowledge transfer that ensures growth for eryone involved. This interconnectedness defines the essence of mentorship—it is not just about individual ogress, but about building a system where each member contributes to the learning of others.

eflecting on my journey, I realize that this mentorship has been one of the most defining experiences of my life. has given me more than just knowledge it has instilled in me a responsibility to contribute, to teach, and to keep e cycle alive. For anyone who aspires to grow in the field of neurosurgery, this mentorship is a testament that ou should never walk alone.

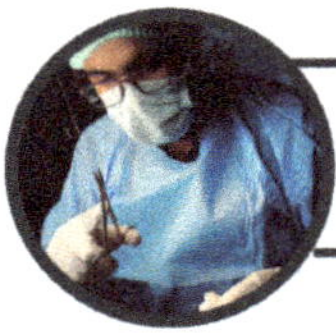

Muntadher H. Almufadhal

In the early stages of my medical school journey, I was a passionate and ambitious student, yet I often found mys unsure of where to begin or how to channel my enthusiasm effectively. I was deeply fascinated by the brain a neurosurgery, frequently immersing myself in the latest research. However, the thought of contributing to the esteemed publications seemed like a distant dream—one I imagined might take at least a decade to achie Remarkably, under the guidance of Dr. Hoz, I managed to accomplish in a single year what I thought would ta ten. I had the extraordinary privilege of participating in more than six high-level research projects and publishi five chapters in prestigious journals. The most thrilling milestone was contributing to a systematic review a meta-analysis before even graduating from medical school.

This incredible transformation in my academic and personal life can be attributed to Dr. Hoz' exceptio mentorship. His approach was nothing short of profound. He had an uncanny ability to discern exactly what ea trainee needed to grow and tailored his guidance accordingly. For me, he recognized a passionate but unstructur drive, and with his mentorship, that passion became a productive force. I went from someone who merely admir scientific research to someone who actively contributed to it. Today, these achievements are not only a source immense pride for me but also for my parents, who now joyfully share my successes with others. It's heartwarmi to see how one person's dedication can instill pride and purpose not just in students but in entire families.

What made this mentorship truly extraordinary was Dr. Hoz' unique personality. He didn't simply act as traditional supervisor; he saw us through a fatherly lens, nurturing us with affection and compassion while holdi us to the highest standards of discipline and excellence. He had an incredible balance of being approachable a supportive while remaining firm and uncompromising when it came to mistakes. This duality refined not only c academic capabilities but also our character. He instilled in us a love for hard work, a deep appreciation for scien and a sense of responsibility that continues to guide us.

The mentorship experience was transformative, not just academically but also personally. It was a rigorous journe requiring countless late nights to fully grasp complex topics. Yet, every challenge was worth it. The results exceeded our expectations, as we emerged from the program not only with tangible achievements but with clari direction, and a profound sense of purpose.

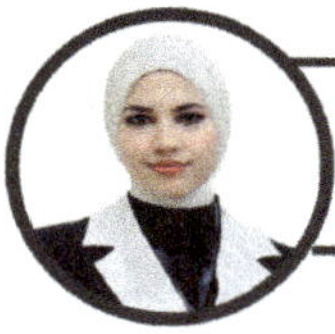

Fatimah Ayad

hey say it's about the journey, not just the goal. In this mentorship, the journey has been just as rewarding as the :stination.

all began when I was a second-year medical student, driven by a growing passion for neuroanatomy. I may not member the exact day I joined this mentorship, but I vividly recall the first time I stepped into an operating room. efore medical school, I had little interest in surgery, but that first day in the OR was an experience beyond my cpectations.

ne day, a friend asked me about the best day of my life. Without hesitation, I mentioned that moment. Many ight not understand how a day in the hospital could be so meaningful, but this mentorship made it possible. The mmunication, the shared passion, and the supportive environment transformed learning into something truly ecial.

his mentorship brought together individuals ranging from second-year students to neurosurgery residents, yet eryone felt involved and valued. Since that day, I have attended many surgeries across different teams and ecialties, but not all experiences were the same. A mentor can either make the OR an unforgettable learning cperience like what Dr. Hoz did or just another routine day.

nlike many programs where students passively observe, this mentorship fostered an interactive and engaging arning environment that made every moment in the OR valuable.

ver the years, this mentorship has been more than just a program; it has been a defining chapter of my medical urney. Beyond clinical exposure, it provided invaluable guidance for those interested in both clinical and :ademic fields. I still remember writing my first research paper and the excitement of every publication that llowed. Being surrounded by like-minded peers and mentor who inspire and guide you makes achieving what ice seemed impossible feel within reach. This experience was not just about theoretical learning—it was about tting an example of the path to follow, gaining hands-on experience, and connecting with some of the best minds the field.

s time passed, this journey gave me confidence and deepened my passion—not only for neurosurgery but also r opportunities I had never imagined. Beyond neurosurgery and research, this mentorship introduced me to minars, presentations, and collaborations with mentors and colleagues from diverse backgrounds—all united by e same passion. These meetings went beyond sharing scientific knowledge; they carried invaluable life lessons. hey also taught me how to present my work effectively and gave me the confidence to stand before an audience. hat confidence later helped me win a research competition among all Iraqi medical colleges—an achievement itside the mentorship but undoubtedly shaped by the skills I developed within it.

his experience has not only shaped my understanding of neurosurgery but has also taught me the true impact of entorship. One day, I hope to contribute to guiding future students, just as I was guided.

ooking back, my second-year self would have never imagined that one decision could have such a lasting impact. ut without a doubt, she would be proud.

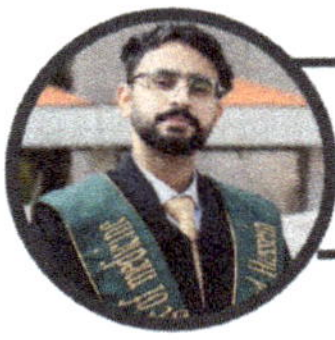

Mahmood H. AlObaidy

Life has an uncanny way of shaping us through experiences that leave indelible marks on our souls. For me, t goal of becoming a neurosurgeon began not with ambition but with profound loss. As a child, I witnessed t deaths of my mother and brother—both due to conditions that could have been treated if there had there been acce to skilled neurosurgical care. At the time, I was too young to fully grasp the gravity of what had happened, but I grew older and understood the circumstances surrounding their passing, I was overcome with shock. Th realization ignited within me a deep desire to dedicate my life to preventing such tragedies for others. It becar clear that I wanted to become a neurosurgeon—not just as a career choice, but as a calling.

Fate, it seems, conspired to guide me toward this goal in ways I never imagined. During my third year of medic school, I encountered Dr. Hoz, whose mentorship would prove transformative. Our meeting felt serendipitous– coincidence so powerful that it almost seemed preordained. From our very first conversation, Dr. Hoz exuc inspiration. He spoke with passion about the intricacies of neurosurgery, shared stories of resilience, and instill in me the belief that no goal is unattainable if pursued with determination. Every interaction with him left inspired, ambitious, and more confident than before. His guidance taught me not only the technical aspects neurosurgery but also the importance of empathy, creativity, and critical thinking in patient care.

Under his mentorship, I embraced opportunities I might otherwise have shied away from. Attending surgeri observing seasoned neurosurgeons, and engaging in thought-provoking discussions opened my eyes to the v possibilities within this field. One particularly pivotal moment in my mentorship journey came when Dr. H offered me an opportunity to participate in writing a neurosurgery book. This marked my very first publicati and it was an incredibly enriching experience. Not only did it deepen my understanding of neuroradiology, bu also honed my skills in academic writing, critical thinking, and collaboration. Working on this project allowed to grow both personally and professionally, and it reinforced the transformative power of mentorship in helpi individuals achieve milestones they once thought was out of reach. Writing about neurosurgery—a subject I on feared was beyond my reach—felt like bridging two worlds: my passion for storytelling and my love for medici

Looking back, I realize that mentorship played a crucial role in my development. Dr. Hoz didn't just teach me; empowered me to think creatively, write boldly, and dream fearlessly. Through his support, I learned that succe isn't achieved alone—it's nurtured through collaboration, encouragement, and trust. Today, as I stand at t beginning of my career, I carry with me not only the lessons of my past but also the unwavering belief that eve challenge can be transformed into an opportunity. The road ahead may be long, but I walk it with purpose, knowi that my journey will honor those I lost and inspire future generations to pursue their goals.

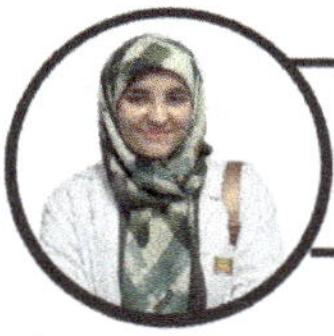

Huda Abdulrazaq

'o and a half years ago, a friend invited me to a mentorship program led by Dr. Hoz. Though I knew little about n or medical research, I was impressed by how the mentorship program guided students into the field.

ter a year of hesitation, I finally asked Dr. Hoz for a research opportunity. Then I witnessed the process of how estions evolve into meaningful studies. I never imagined publishing a research paper in an international journal a medical student, but the Hoz mentorship made it possible.

enever we asked Dr. Hoz something, he would say, let's turn this into research. His continuous encouragement shes us to explore complex challenges and find answers through science. But this experience was more than just iting research papers. I learned to be bold, think critically, and question everything. Dr. Hoz showed me that owledge isn't just something to memorize—it's something we can create. This realization changed how I proach medicine and gave me the confidence to contribute to scientific progress.

z mentorship program also strengthened my communication, teamwork, and patient care skills. More portantly, it showed me the power of mentorship as I thought learning was a solo journey, but I now understand t having a great mentor makes all the difference.

matter where my medical career takes me—whether neurosurgery or another field—the lessons I've learned l stay with me. This experience didn't just teach me about research; it shaped the way I think, learn, and work h others.

oking back, I feel incredibly grateful to be one of the fortunate students who had the mentorship woven into ir daily lives. This experience has shaped me in ways I never imagined, allowing me to see medicine from a ole new perspective. I witnessed diverse opinions, met people from different backgrounds, and saw them all ne together in pursuit of science.

ould not be the person I am today without the impact of the mentorship and Dr. Hoz guidance. I will forever be nkful for this opportunity. I accomplished things I never thought I was capable of—tackling complex and llenging topics that once seemed beyond my reach. I worked on difficult subjects, such as systematic reviews middle cerebral artery aneurysms, a field I never imagined I could contribute to. This journey showed me how I could push myself and how much this mentorship helped me grow.

ese years of my life have been incredibly meaningful because of the mentorship program experience. I will never get the moment Dr. Hoz told me I needed to work on myself. At that time, I was hungry to learn, driven to prove, and he always believed in me. I am proud of how far I have come, and I will always be thankful for Hoz ntorship program and for Dr. Hoz continuous support.

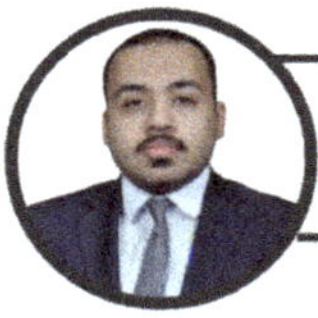

Mostafa H. Algabri

I thank God for this path and for everything that has shaped me into who I am today. This journey, with all its tr and challenges, has defined my existence. Without these relentless efforts, I would not recognize myself; they the very essence of my being.

I am fully aware that this path is arduous, at times seemingly impossible. Yet, my unwavering faith in God's di plan reassures me. The burning desire within me is not a coincidence, nor is it meaningless. It was planted in heart for a purpose, and that purpose is what fuels my perseverance. No matter how difficult the road may see will continue forward, trusting that every step is part of something greater than I can comprehend.

I studied at the College of Medicine at the University of Baghdad, becoming the first member of my famil pursue a medical degree. I had always felt a deep and persistent desire to understand neuroscience, a passion led me toward medical research despite the many challenges and obstacles I encountered along the way.

In my final year, I met Dr. Hoz during an online meeting. He was truly exceptional, someone with a commanc presence who always knew exactly what to say and when to say it. That encounter was not a mere coincidenc became a turning point that reshaped my academic and professional path.

His primary focus was helping students and providing them with opportunities to engage in medical resea particularly in the field of neurosurgery. Inspired by his enthusiasm and support, I felt an overwhelming driv enter this field. I started working with him on several research projects while simultaneously preparing for United States Medical Licensing Exams (USMLE). His support extended far beyond research; he became a me who guided me through my studies and even influenced some of my major life decisions. His presence mark pivotal shift in my journey. Today, three years later, I fully recognize that knowing him was a defining mome my life. I now have 15 published research papers, with five more in progress. I have also completed my USM exams, unlocking new opportunities I had never imagined.

I still remember the day I first spoke to him about my desire to enter the world of research. I was hesitant, fi with self-doubt due to my lack of prior experience. Yet, he welcomed me with open arms, without hesitatio skepticism. He patiently taught me the fundamentals of scientific writing, reviewing every piece I wrote, correc it, and guiding me through every detail with unwavering dedication.

I recall his words: *"What is done for the sake of God will always grow."* It wasn't just a phrase; it was a princ he lived by. He didn't just guide me. He helped me publish four research papers, with my name listed as the author. His support went beyond research; he remained in constant contact, checking in on me whenev disappeared for a while, always asking about my progress and how far I had come in achieving my goals.

He always addressed in a paternal tone. It was a genuine expression of scientific mentorship and a sincere de to see us succeed and grow.

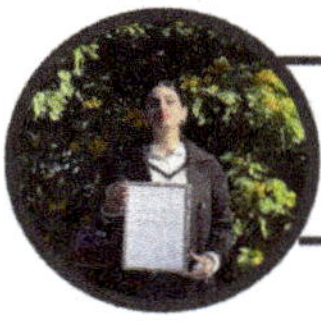

Haneen A. Salih

ve been captivated by the intricate workings of the mind from a young age, driven by a burning curiosity to ıravel the mysteries of the brain. Growing up in Iraq, this passion often felt like a silent yearning—something too nbitious to name aloud. Yet, pursuing this dream seemed impossible in a country where neuroscience as a field nonexistent. Entering this field—let alone gaining hands-on experience—seemed out of reach, until I found the oz Neurosurgery Mentorship. This program became the sole opportunity that allowed me to step into the world f the brain.

nder the guidance of Dr. Hoz, I delved into topics like neuroanatomy, neuroradiology, and research ethodologies. What began as an academic pursuit soon evolved into a life-changing journey, reshaping my terests and aspirations in ways I could never have imagined.

ne of the most profound experiences of this mentorship was in the operating room, where I had the rare pportunity to observe and assist in a craniotomy. One case that left an indelible mark on me involved the removal f a deep precentral gyrus cavernoma—an area critical for motor control. The use of functional mapping and traoperative neurophysiological monitoring to identify anatomical landmarks and preserve motor function was othing short of astonishing. In that moment, I felt both humbled and electrified—a quiet voice inside me said, This is where I belong." It made me realize the practical significance of research and innovation and how nowledge can directly translate into clinical settings to improve patients' quality of life.

ach experience in the operating room deepened my appreciation for the magnificence of the human brain—not st as an organ, but as the very essence of what gives life meaning. Witnessing the delicate precision of eurosurgery and the surgical management of neurological disorders left me in awe of the brain's beauty and omplexity. These moments reshaped my perspective on science and research, igniting a passion for bridging the ap between basic science and real-world applications.

eyond the OR, the mentorship opened doors to research I never thought I'd walk through. I learned to critically ppraise literature, design studies, and write academic papers. I was exposed to a global standard of scientific inking and became a co-author on peer-reviewed publications—a milestone I once believed was years away. Not ng ago, I struggled to access scientific papers—now, I am contributing to them.

ne Hoz Neurosurgery Mentorship didn't just teach me; it reshaped how I think. It was more than an educational xperience—it was a lifeline. It showed me that passion and determination, when paired with the right guidance, an overcome even the most daunting barriers. It instilled not only knowledge and skill but also the confidence to elieve I belonged in this field.

his journey showed me that mentorship doesn't just shape careers—it transforms communities. In places like aq, where access to specialized training is limited, such programs are life-changing. They empower aspiring inicians and scientists to lead and innovate where it's needed most. I am no longer just a student fascinated by e brain—I am a neuroscientist in the making, determined to give back to the field that has given me so much. nd for that, I will always be grateful.

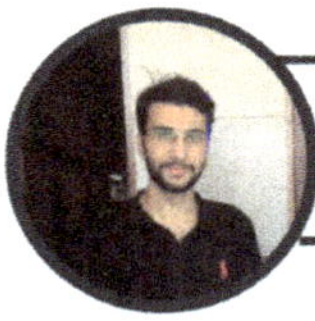

Jaafar Abdulwahid

Nature is magnificent for countless reasons, Nature continuous process of refinement and transformation. As observer and learner, you inevitably arrive at the concept of innovation, a fundamental principle that shapes life will return to this concept shortly.

I've graduated from medical school recently, but back in the early years of my medical education, I was captivat by the extraordinary complexity of the brain and nervous system. Neuroscience was not just a subject I studied was a field that sparked my imagination and curiosity, I dealt with it as something futuristic. That interest led r one day to attend an online Zoom meeting of the "HOZ Mentorship Program", which started with 3-4 hours brain firing. From the very first moments you can conclude that was not just another lecture, it was somethi innovative and uniquely engaging.

Over three years since that meeting with all the experiences and feelings I have faced, now I can summarize it w the concept of innovation. Exposing to different levels of experiences, ranging from attending neurosurger (neurovascular, neuro-oncology, endovascular surgeries), engaging with neurosurgical cases, listening international guests, and encouraging mentees to think critically and contribute ideas that shape the mentorsh itself. That is a place where the mentees grow in different ways, all find part interests them whether in the field neurosurgery or beyond.

There is always something new to gain, scientific knowledge, philosophical insights, personal development, or ne perspectives. Listening to the experiences of neurosurgeons from different cultural and professional backgroun interacting with their ideas, and absorbing their advice that summarizes professional and personal life will mak change in mentality and reshape the way I think about the future as a human and neurosurgeon in this world.

This mentorship program reminds me of how nature nurtures growth, a fertile ground where seeds grow a flourish smoothly. That's also for a student in this mentorship. And that, to me, is true innovation. Innovati mentorship is to create a life-changing environment for those students in a 'War-torn area' when their dreams ha been suppressed for a long time. Free from limitations and develop confidence in their abilities and potential.

HOZ Neurosurgery Mentorship is a paradigm. The greatest gift to the new generation is not just knowledge bu framework to elevate them beyond the starting line. And that's what have been provided by the establisher of H Mentorship Program, a true mentorship cultivates growth and transformation. Shaping the road for us as mente to push neurosurgery in our country and benefit our people and the world. With that been said all thanks to gr human and mentor Dr Samer Hoz.

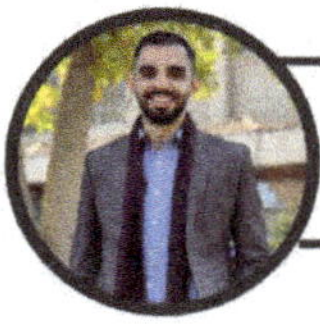

Younus M. Al-Khazaali

I was asked to choose a suitable title for my experience within this mentorship program, this quote will ummarize it all:

f you are the smartest person in the room, then you are in the wrong room."

never imagined that a single mentorship program could redefine my perspective on neurosurgery and reshape my pirations. Coming from a country where neurosurgery was often viewed as an undefeatable challenge, it was ually seen as a field filled with risks rather than possibilities. The lack of resources, the overwhelming sponsibilities, and the societal obstacles made it one of the least pursued specialties in Iraq. However, my journey ok an unexpected turn when I joined Dr. Hoz's neurosurgery mentorship program.

was always fascinated by the human brain, even before getting accepted into medical school, this complex and rgeous creation was always a mystery that I wanted to explore. However, the path to this mystery seemed unclear me because of the obstacles that I mentioned earlier. On top of that, my path was lacking an essential part, a entor, which is something that I wasn't aware of since most of the doctors I met till that moment used to follow e common pathway which was to graduate from medical school, finish the post-graduate years, then competing get into the safest and easiest specialty in our country without considering other essential factors that should fluence their choice. One of the most important factors in my opinion is passion, this aspect which is mostly glected when choosing a specialty here because of the same obstacles. However, after enrolling in the Hoz eurosurgery mentorship, a lot of these standards were changed.

om the very first meeting, I was captivated by the depth of knowledge and passion shared by my mentor. His ility to navigate the complexities of neurosurgery, leadership, and teaching in a setting with limited resources as nothing short of inspiring. I was no longer just a student learning the fundamentals of medicine—I was itnessing firsthand how dedication and innovation could overcome even the toughest challenges. Shadowing rgeries, engaging in discussions, and interacting with like-minded mentees broadened my perspective. eurosurgery was no longer an impossible feat but rather a calling that demanded perseverance and vision

ne of the most valuable lessons I gained from this mentorship was that limitations are often self-imposed. roughout the program, I met students who, like me, initially doubted their ability to pursue such a demanding ecialty. But with each passing week, we learned to replace doubt with curiosity, fear with determination and entually each one of us discovered a hidden talent that was hidden inside them. I discovered that flexibility is the ckbone of any great neurosurgeon, and mentorship provides the compass to navigate this challenging yet warding path.

nis experience was more than just an introduction to a medical specialty—it was a transformation. It instilled in e a profound sense of purpose, a belief that despite the hardships, pursuing neurosurgery in a low-resource setting not only possible but essential, not only this but following this path in such circumstances and excelling in it will shape the future of this country. The mentorship I received not only shaped my career aspirations but also engthened my confidence in facing obstacles head-on. I will always be grateful for the opportunity to be part of program that illuminated a path I once thought was out of reach.

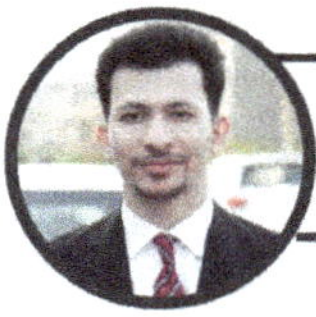

Sajjad Ghanim Al-Badri

Some opportunities redefine your path in ways you never anticipated. When I first joined the mentorship progra I had zero knowledge about research and publications. I was eager to learn but unsure where to begin. The wo of research seemed distant, something that required years of expertise before making any meaningful contributi However, this mentorship changed everything. Two years later, I now have over 45 publications—a transformati I never imagined possible.

Looking back, I believe that joining this mentorship was the most important step in my journey toward masteri research. It wasn't just about learning how to conduct studies or publish papers; it was about developing a mind of curiosity, perseverance, and collaboration. Dr. Hoz's guidance was invaluable, not only in providing knowled but also in shaping the way I approached academic work. His mentorship instilled in me the confidence to take challenges that once seemed far beyond my capabilities.

One of the most remarkable aspects of this experience was the collaborative environment within the mentorsh Research is often perceived as a solitary endeavor, but I quickly realized that meaningful progress happens throu teamwork. The team dynamics within the program taught me how to work seamlessly with others, combini different strengths to achieve something greater than any individual effort. I learned how to contribute effective give and receive constructive feedback, and recognize that every role—no matter how small—plays a vital part the success of a research project.

There were moments of struggle, times when I doubted whether I could keep up with the fast pace of research. I in those moments, I found support from my mentor and my peers. The mentorship didn't just equip me w technical skills; it provided a community that fostered growth. Every research project was an opportunity to le something new. I learned that persistence is just as important as intelligence and that failures were not setbacks steppingstones to improvement.

Perhaps the most surprising part of this journey was realizing how much I enjoyed research. Initially, I saw it as academic requirement—something necessary for career advancement. But as I became more involved, I discove the excitement of exploring unanswered questions, the satisfaction of uncovering new insights, and the pride contributing to scientific knowledge. Research was no longer just a skill; it became a passion.

Through this experience, I've come to appreciate that success in research isn't just about individual knowledge it's about teamwork, mentorship, and the willingness to step into the unknown. This mentorship didn't just tea me how to publish; it taught me how to grow, collaborate, and push beyond my own limits. It showed me that right guidance and the right team can make the impossible seem achievable. I now approach every challenge w the mindset that there is always a way forward, always something to learn, and always a team to lean on.

Reflecting on my journey, I am grateful for the opportunity to be part of this mentorship. It has shaped my acader career in ways I never expected, and I know that the lessons I've learned here will stay with me for a lifetime.

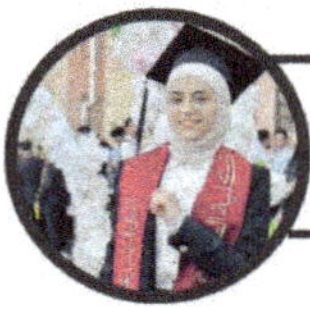

Zainab Abdualmurtafie

: should never walk alone. This is one of the fundamentals that I learned from Dr. Hoz in this program, ognizing the benefits of networking and guidance for junior doctors, making it crystal clear how much of an pact these supporting programs have in shaping us to be successful medical professionals, leaders, and future ntors ourselves. Till today I remember first meeting Dr. Hoz; I was carrying mixed emotions from being anxious l afraid of making mistakes or doing something wrong to being delighted to finally meet him in person. I traveled rying all these emotions from where I lived, to Baghdad, about 341 kilometers away.

e second obstacle was being a female traveling this far to attend such a program in another city. It's uncommon our culture but being raised in a family where both parents are physicians and knowing how much knowledge l confidence I could gain from this program, they approved it. Other obstacles like attending college, work, and sonal commitment were in the way as well. Despite all of this, I went through, and I am grateful to my brave ıng version of myself for taking this unique adventure. This was a big step for me, for someone who had been fering from imposter syndrome for more than 4 years of medical school and thought any success I had was due uck rather than my abilities and hard work. I never felt glad for all the achievements that I made, and there was vays something missing, I wasn't good enough for sure, and there was no room for any kind of mistakes.

ile shadowing the team I didn't feel the time passing while observing Dr. Hoz in the operating room and ergency department and how he led the team, gave instructions to each one on how they work in such harmony, igned each member specific roles and responsibilities, and guided in an individualized and achievable plan hin the needed period. Recognizing the strengths and weak points in each member and providing actionable dback that focuses on both while pointing out opportunities for improvement. I was amazed about all the mwork principles they have, how to address and talk to each member with each mentee being responsible for /her actions, what and when to ask questions, how to respond concerning. To be honest, I was so jealous of my er peers who were situated in Baghdad, as they had a chance to meet him and the team in person more often. spite the short period of meeting Dr. Hoz and the geographical distance. Dr. Hoz creates a communication plan h multiple ways of connection, he was open to adjusting timelines and exploring alternative approaches if ded to continue being on track.

ekly and monthly Zoom meetings, national and international, with post-presentation conversations, which were most interesting parts, discussing what went wrong and right and how to avoid it in the future. Here comes the portance of technology that simplifies connection and smooths workflow .Dr. Hoz trained us to respect the time hose who must listen to us, be brief, be ethical, and handle criticism from him with dignity and respect. I was lled with the opportunity to be part of a few articles that were published by the team as well.

ou rise by raising the people around you" was the first thing I heard from Dr. Hoz, and to this day I work by it. moral visions and his boundless enthusiasm are captivating and outstanding, making us amazed every time. bracing these fundamental values will not only create a supportive and effective training environment but will integrate the main ethical considerations that must be constructed in every doctor.

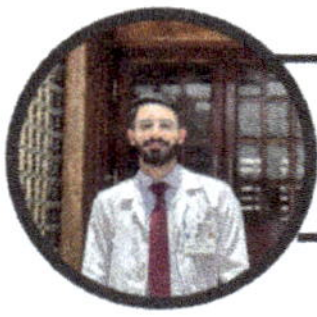

Saleh Abdulkareem Saleh

I believe that everything in life happens for a reason, and some events can take us far beyond what we hope expected. From my point of view, mentorship simply means relationship plus guidance. At the HOZ mentor program, I found more than just that. It was not just an academic exposure but a life-changing experience. T more insightful, I will put my experience into three levels.

First the educational and scientific perspective; as a medical student who has a growing passion to learn and st more about brains this mentorship was a really great opportunity to be exposed to this field from inside. Learn more about the neuroanatomy that we have just studied at the medical college and its true significance in e step in every neurosurgery is something rewarding. I can still remember when Dr. Hoz teaches us the pre-opera anatomy of interest, then guides us during the operation room through every step to make us more oriented on field.

My first experience in theater as an observer student was a patient who underwent a clipping for poste communicating artery aneurysm. It was very interesting—at least for me—and still vivid in my memory wher finally got the clipping step, and it was successful. Watching this kind of operation is inspiring, and it beco more delightful when our patients get better. Furthermore, seeing the smile on the patient's face and sensing family's gratitude and warm feelings is something very rewarding.

During those case study periods, I got more oriented about the scientific complexity of the neurosurgery fi however, within those complexities, Dr. Hoz guides us on how to study these subjects, providing us with required resources and sharing his experiences, which make it easier to get the most impact from these teac sessions.

The second perspective is the guiding and behaving part; it is crucial to learn how to act with peers and with o medical professionals and how to approach and deal with patients appropriately. Dr. Hoz was a real exampl those situations. I used to observe how he acted and communicated with team members. Good communica makes the work dynamic easier and goal-directed. For instance, during operations, I watch the whole team v flawlessly for many hours like a beehive, where each individual knows exactly their role and what to do and to do it, all these efforts guided for the patient's best interest.

The last part of this mentorship I consider vital is the growth and networking; I used to have an interest in resea so at this space I got many opportunities to be part of various projects, including writing research pap participating in books as a chapter author, and leading research teams. These activities kept me active and in cor with many kind people who share common goals. I consider my experience during this program is life shifting support and the guidance I got is crucial and add more to my personality. I believe this mentorship gave something I will forever be grateful for, and I hope to follow the line in supporting following generations some

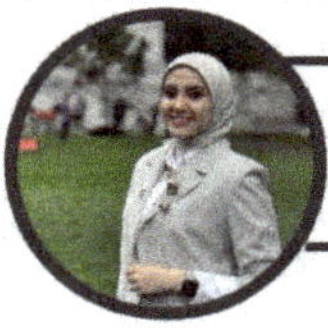

Saja Amer Albanaa

ıe earlier steps you take in life often pave the way for your future. I joined Hoz mentorship program six years ;o, an experience that continues to influence my career to this day. I look back on it with immense gratitude. The ost impressive aspect about it is, despite the limited-resources country that it took place in, Dr. Hoz did his best give us a perfect exposure to neurosurgery.

ne of the most memorable aspects was the hands-on training. I can still recall the excitement of using a surgical ill to perform a burr hole on a dead sheep skull and how we craved our names over an egg without puncturing its ell, to learn the delicacy in the field.

elieve this kind of mentorships is what the world need. Specifically, it can help students in deciding their future edical specialty, bridge the gap between academic studies and hospital settings, and help in networking for a ture collaboration.

lways owe this experience the gratitude as it has impacted my career significantly. And for any project to succeed must have a great leader. Through Hoz Mentorship Program, Dr. Hoz proved his keenness and dedication to not st be considered as a great leader but a life-long mentor. Throughout the years I always seek Dr. Hoz advice and are with him any milestone I achieve. Moreover, I co-authored many articles with my mentorship colleagues and ade some friendships along the way.

vould encourage anyone to join this program. It is an opportunity not just to gain knowledge and skills but to rm connections that will support and inspire you throughout your career.

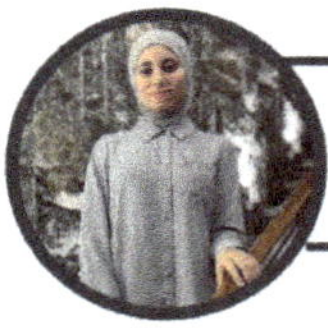

Naba Ghazwan

My story with neurosurgery might sound a little different. I was in high school when I used to spend summ holidays playing video games, and a neuroscientist was the main character in one of them. I was fascinated everything related to the brain at that time and continued my studies to enter medical school. This love neurology only increased during my second year of medical school when I studied neuroanatomy. During that tin I saw an announcement for the Hoz mentorship from a friend and enrolled immediately, as I needed someone tell me more about this specialty. With my first meeting in the mentorship with Dr. Samer Hoz, I realized this what I needed—a mentor to guide me and Dr. Hoz was truly the best mentor ever, turning my fascination w neurosurgery into something tangible.

Through the mentorship, the most precious thing I learned is teamwork. Dr. Hoz gave us tasks and research proje to work on as a team, and everyone did his or her best to achieve the best results. Another thing Dr. Hoz gave the opportunity to attend surgeries with him, but for some reason, I could not attend any. So I eagerly awaited otl mentees' feedback after each surgery they attended, and I searched and learned more about anything new I he from their feedback.

Something we are not familiar with as undergraduates: every idea in the mentorship is welcomed, every though appreciated, and could be the beginning of something big turned into an article, a chapter in a book, an internatio presentation, and more. This is considered an achievement for the idea's owner and a benefit for other mentees.

From the mentorship, I was given an opportunity to participate in research projects, and I achieved one of dreams; to have publications before graduating from college. I absolutely could not have done that without Dr. H support and other mentees' hard work.

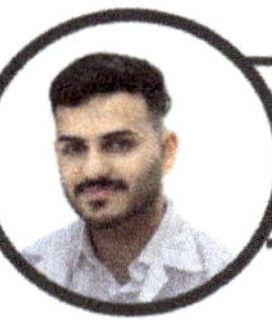

Mohammedbaqer Ghuraibawi

ıe journey of learning is never easy; it requires dedication, perseverance, intent commitment to knowledge. etting a small piece of science needs all the power in life. Investing a lifetime in the pursuit of science often yields ıly fragments of understanding, making every small achievement valuable. At the outset, uncertainty can cloud e path, with every decision seeming weighty and every challenge appearing daunting. However, no one should ıvigate this journey alone. Having a good mentor to guide represents a defining factor in shaping academic and ofessional growth. Choosing the right mentor not provide knowledge only but also cultivates the to be a good ɛcision maker and enhance confidence and resilience. Fortunately, I have met Dr. Samer Hoz, who gave me the ɛperience of this firsthand through his mentorship program, his efforts were the main cause to support and insight ı instrumental role in my development in neurosurgery.

uring my first years in medical school, I always dreamed of being a successful neurosurgeon and a researcher, I as filled with ambition and a deep passion for research and neurosurgery but lacked a clear vision of the right rection. Like most medical students, I felt overwhelmed by the complexities of the field that I love, struggling to ıart a course to my goals. My enthusiasm for learning was associated with self-doubt, and always questioned hether my aspirations were beyond reach. All these thoughts and situations changed when I had the privilege of ɛing mentored by Dr. Samer Hoz. He is a great mentor by all means; his approach extends beyond academics.

ıe lessons that I learned in Hoz's mentorship program cannot be counted, He taught me not only science but also hics, communication skills, work proficiency, commitment, critical thinking, creativity, and many other critical ırts of my journey. Dr. Hoz opened the window of neurosurgery and research for me, he encouraged me to seek ıt opportunities. His steadfast belief in my potential instilled in me a new level of confidence, allowing me to plore research, refine my skills, and gain invaluable hands-on experience that significantly influenced my ademic journey. Among most of neurosuegeons, Dr. Hoz has been a model of leadership, perseverance, and ofessionalism. His passion and dedication have inspired me to build strong basics in my journey to become a ccessful neurosurgeon, I always dream of having his commit to lifelong learning and continuous self-ıprovement.

ɛflecting on this experience, I now realize the profound impact that mentorship has had on my journey. entorship was not merely about acquiring knowledge, it was a journey about discovering my strengths, veloping my mindset, and overcoming self-doubt. Under the guidance of Dr. Hoz, I had a lot of opportunities d insights that most students cannot gain, his guidance has provided me with a clear sense of direction. I cannot more grateful for his unwavering support and belief in my abilities and developing them.

ıe lessons I have learned from Dr. Hoz will be the foundation for my future endeavors, and his impact on my ırney is something I will always cherish. I am forever appreciative of the knowledge, inspiration, and couragement he has provided, as they have been instrumental in shaping the person I am today.

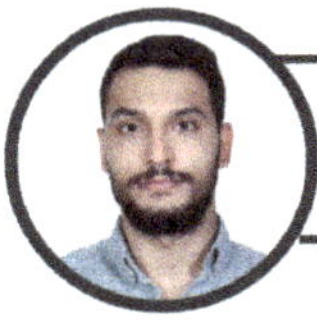

Mustafa Shukur

Some passions begin quietly like a spark you do not yet realize is a flame.
When I reached my final year of medical school, I knew I loved neurosurgery; however, I didn't fully understa why. My affection for this field was unformed—raw and uninformed, without a clear direction. That all chang when I joined the HOZ Neurosurgery Mentorship Program.
Dr. Hoz welcomed me into the world of neurosurgery with open arms, and ever since then, something within has shifted. The Neurosurgery Teaching Hospital was no longer a place to visit in order to learn; it was hon Occasionally, I would shed the stress of exams and head to the hospital, where the energy soothed me; I felt lik belonged there. One of the standout moments in my experience was watching an aneurysmal clipping procedu I witnessed the careful preparation, the pre-operative discussion, and the focus of the operating team. It was first time I truly grasped the weight and elegance of neurosurgery; it was then that I realized—profoundly a clearly—that this was the path I wanted to follow for the rest of my life.
That mentorship was more than just clinical exposure—it changed the way I saw myself, my goals, and what ki of doctor I wanted to become. In the lab, I was trained by Dr. Hoz on surgical microscopes and performed precisi activities using loops. Those were not just technical skill training, I was taught to think, move, and make decisio like surgeons do. Each session in the lab made me more focused and passionate.
These memories are significant milestones in my journey, moments of growth, teamwork and inspiration. I lo back at them as special memories and the foundation of my future. They are sketched in my mind like vivid imag —scrubbing in with the team, listening to pre-operative discussions, flipping through pages in the lab, and feeli for the first time, that I was in the right place.
That mentorship didn't just improve my skills; it shaped my identity. I learned to love neurosurgery not just a discipline but as a purpose. I will always be grateful to Dr. Hoz for creating an environment that helped me disco that purpose and guided me during one of the most crucial times of my life.

Section 3: Reflections and Future Directions

Conclusion: Shaping the Future of Neurosurgery through a Lasting Mentorship Legacy

As this book draws to a close, we reflect on the journey that brought us here. The stories, the challenges, and the triumphs that have defined the Hoz Neurosurgery Mentorship Program. Through the pages of You Should NEVER Walk Alone, we have shared a vision of mentorship that transcends the traditional teacher-student relationship. It is a vision of collaboration, of shared growth, and of creating a legacy that continues long after the first lesson is taught.

This book was never about recording the successes of our mentorship program but was to serve as a living model of what mentorship can achieve. This journey, from the operating theatre to the lecture hall, in personal development to professional excellence, has shown that mentorship is not a one-way street. It's a partnership wherein a mentor and mentee grow, learn, and inspire each other.

As we look toward the future, the impact of mentorship becomes even more evident. The mentees who have passed through this program are not just students. They are future leaders, innovators, and mentors themselves. This book has highlighted the transformative power of mentorship, especially in resource-limited settings, where the challenges are many, but the drive to succeed is even greater. These lessons learned transcend neurosurgery to touch on any field in a way that will bring structured, compassionate, and sustainable mentorship programs to the forefront. Whether you are a mentor desiring to guide the next generation or a seeking student, the principles in this book are naturally universal.

The Hoz Neurosurgery Mentorship Program is more than a project. It is a legacy. And while this book may have reached its conclusion, the story of mentorship continues. Each mentee who walks away from this program does so with the tools, confidence, and support to walk their own path. Never alone, but always supported by the knowledge that they are part of something greater. Ultimately, we want this book to be-a reflection for us and an inspiration for others-to start their journey. At the core of it all, mentorship is walking together, sharing wisdom, and building a future whereby all may thrive. Therefore, even as we walk on, remember you are never to walk alone-because that's where greatness was achieved: when we walk together.

List of Publications

Articles

1. Ajaj, Seraj, Saber Zafarshamspour, Teeba A. Al-Ageely, Mohammedbaqer Ghuraibawi, Ahmed Muthana, Mayur Sharma, and Samer S. Hoz. "Rituals and superstitions in neurosurgery." Surgical Neurology International 16 (2025): 15.
2. Abdalridha, Rokaya H., Ahmed Muthana, Furqan R. Hassooni, Noor Al-Saadi, Arwa Jader, and Samer S. Hoz. "Distal middle cerebral artery aneurysms: What non-neurosurgeons need to know." Surgical Neurology International 16, no. 49 (2025): 1.
3. Muthana, Ahmed, Haneen A. Salih, Mubarak Jolayemi Mustapha, Hussein Salih Abed, Alkawthar M. Abdulsada, Aktham O. Al-Khafaji, Zainab KA Alaraji, Mayur Sharma, and Samer S. Hoz. "Trigeminal nerve palsy associated with intracranial aneurysms: Scoping review." Surgical Neurology International 16, no. 38 (2025): 1.
4. Samer S. Hoz, Paolo Palmisciano, Ahmed Muthana, Edward J. Doyle III1, Mark D. Johnson, Mustafa Ismail, Jonathan A. Forbes, Charles J. Prestigiacomo, Ravi Samy, Mario Zuccarello, Norberto Andaluz. A standalone minimally invasive presigmoid retrolabyrinthine suprameatal approach: A cadaveric morphometric study. 28-Feb-2025;16:68
5. Samer S. Hoz, Paolo Palmisciano, Mustafa Ismail, Ahmed Muthana, Edward J. Doyle, Mark D. Johnson, Jonathan A. Forbes, Charles J. Prestigiacomo, Ravi Samy, Mario Zuccarello, Norberto Andaluz. Minimally invasive presigmoid retrolabyrinthine suprameatal approach (PRSA): A cadaveric study for accessing premeatal anterior inferior cerebellar artery (AICA) aneurysms. 04-Oct-2024;15:364
6. Samer S. Hoz, Li Ma, Ahmed Muthana, Mahmood Falah Al-Zaidy, Fatimah Oday Ahmed, Mustafa Ismail, Rachel C. Jacobs, Prateek Agarwal, Alhamza R. Al-Bayati, Raul G. Nogueira, Michael J. Lang, Bradley A. Gross1. Cranial nerve palsies and intracranial aneurysms: A narrative review of patterns and outcomes. Surgical Neurology International. 09-Aug-2024;15:277.
7. Atallah O, Muthana A, Sanker V, Wawi O, Samer S. Hoz. Mapping the circle of Trolard: A holistic view of its role in neurosurgical practice, anatomical perspectives and clinical applications. Brain and Spine. 2024 Mar 23:102789.

8. Algabri MH, Delawan M, Sharma M, Al-Hilfi MS, Almufadhal MH, Shaker NM, Abdualmurttafie ZI, Ismail M, Andaluz N, Samer S. Hoz. Residual brain AVMs after surgical resection: A literature review of causes and treatment considerations. World Neurosurgery: X. 2024 Mar 21:100366.
9. Ismail M, Matti WE, Kadhum HJ, Taha AM, Mustafa MK, Samer S. Hoz. Gravitational bullet injuries: Unique insights for further investigations. Romanian Neurosurgery. 2024 Mar 15:78-80.
10. Alsubaihawi ZA, Muthana A, Kareem ZM, Ahmed FO, Algburi HA, Al-Khazaal YM, Atallah O, Ismail M, Samer S. Hoz. Posterior auricular artery: Anatomical variations and neurosurgical applications. Romanian Neurosurgery. 2024 Mar 15:81-6.
11. Al-Baider R, Muthana A, Hassan SF, Ahmed FO, Hadi RT, Atallah O, Ismail M, Samer S. Hoz. Supratrochlear artery: Anatomy, variations and neurosurgical applications. Romanian Neurosurgery. 2024 Mar 15:90-3.
12. Ismail M, Al-Qaraghuli AK, Al-Badri SG, Samer S. Hoz. The status of nanoneusurgery investigated. Romanian Neurosurgery. 2024 Mar 15:117-20.
13. Alaraji ZA, Atallah O, Alaraji ZA, Al-Badri SG, Ismail M, Samer S. Hoz. Potential psychological responses in patients who underwent MRI scanning. Romanian Neurosurgery. 2024 Mar 15:87-9.
14. Alfawares Y, Ismail M, Ramanathan VP, Andaluz N, Samer S. Hoz. A case that encapsulates the challenges of being a neurosurgeon in war-torn countries: Perspectives from Iraq. Surgical Neurology International. 2024;15(46):1.
15. Daniela Ramírez-Castillo, Zainab K. A. Alaraji, Daniela Marcela Torres Llinás, Huber Padilla-Zambrano, María Sofia Calle Palmett, Samer S. Hoz. Delays and misdiagnosis of aneurysmal subarachnoid hemorrhage: the impact of socioeconomic barriers. Surgical Neurology International. May 2024.
16. Mubarak J. Mustapha, Ahmed Muthana, Ahmad O. Sulaiman, Samer S. Hoz. Enhancing medical education experience through community-based experience and services. Surgical Neurology International. June 2024.
17. Muhammad Kashif, Ahmed Muthana, Abdullah M. Al-Qudah, Samer S. Hoz. the influence of artificial intelligence on neurological surgery and patient outcome. Surgical Neurology International. June 2024.

18. Ali M. Neamah, Mustafa Ismail, Aktham O. Al- Khafaji, Saja A. Albanaa, Sajjad G. Al-Badri, Almutasimbellah K. Etaiwi, Mays S. A. Ahmed, Mahmood F. Al-Zaidy, Samer S. Hoz. Neurosurgical management of posterior communicating artery aneurysmal perforators. Technical note through two case examples. Romanian Neurosurgery. June 2024.
19. Hagar A. Algburi, Mustafa Ismail, Tabarek M. Al- Nuaimi, Zainab T. Alzeyadi, Jafar M. Sabbar, Ahmed K. Al-Kishawi, Rania H. Al-Taie, Mahmood F. Al-Zaidy, Mohammed A. Alrawi, Samer S. Hoz. Configurational changes of ruptured intracranial aneurysms at the window between pre-operative CTA and the definite clipping surgery. Romanian Neurosurgery. June 2024.
20. Mostafa H. Algabri, Ali Adnan, Asmaa H. AL-Sharee, Sajjad G. Al-Badri, Rania H. Al-Taie, Mustafa Ismail, Samer S. Hoz. Variation in optic recess angle with optic chiasm position. Imaging characteristics of 140 cases. Romanian Neurosurgery. June 2024.
21. Muhammad Kashif, Ahmed Muthana, Abdullah M. Al-Qudah, Samer S. Hoz. the hindrance of matching into neurosurgery from doctors of osteopathic-medicine perspective. Surgical Neurology International. July 2024.
22. Oday Atallah, MD, Gianluca Scalia, MD, Mohammed A. Azab, MD, Ahmed Muthana, MD, Omar Wawi, MD, Vivek Sanker, MBBS, Almutasimbellah K. Etaiwi, MD, Samer S. Hoz, MD. The Role of Precentral Cerebellar Vein in Neurosurgery: An In-depth Review of Anatomy, Implications, and Risks. Brain and Spine. July 2024.
23. Mustafa Ismail, Ali Al-Shalchy, Younus M. Al-Khazaali, Abdelilah Lahmar, Liam V. Goldman, Mostafa H. Algabri, Danisha Kumar, Paolo Palmisciano, Samer S. Hoz. Perioperative blood transfusion management in surgical resection of intracranial meningiomas: A meta-analysis. Surgical Neurology International. July 2024.
24. Teeba A. Al-Ageely, Mustafa Ismail, Zinah A. Alaraji, Jaafar Abdulwahid, Fatima Ayad, Huda Jaafar, Awfa Aktham, Hayder R. Salih, Samer Hoz. Planning a sustainable neurosurgery mentorship program in a war-torn country: experience from Iraq. Chinese Neurosurgical Journal. August 2024.
25. Mubarak Jolayemi J. Mustapha, Ahmed Muthana, James Adedoyin, Samer S. Hoz. Nurturing neurosurgical dreams – Overcoming challenges for medical students in resource-limited settings globally. Surgical Neurology International. August 2024.

26. Mustafa Ismail, Ahmed Muthana, Teeba A. Al-Ageely, Fatimah Oday Ahmed, Rania H. Al-Taie, Aktham O. Al-Khafaji, Mahmood F. Al-Zaidy, Hayder R. Salih, Mohammed A. Alrawi, Awfa Aktham, Hosam Al-Jehani, Samer S. Hoz. Teleproctoring in therapeutic neurointervention: Experience from Iraq-Saudi Arabia collaboration. Surgical Neurology International. August 2024.
27. Sama S. Albairmani, Ahmed Muthana, Tabarek F. Mohammed, Mahmood F. Al-Zaidy, Oday Atallah, Ahmed Aljuboori, Zaid Aljuboori, Norberto Andaluz, Samer S. Hoz. Combined presigmoid approach: A literature review. Surgical Neurology International. September 2024.
28. Mohamed R. Emara, Alkawthar M. Abdulsada, Abdulaziz S. Alayyaf, Hussein A. Baban, Hala A. Al-Hchaimi, Mustafa Ismail, Samer S. Hoz. Ambient Wing Cistern: History, Anatomy, Imaging and Approaches: An Overview. World Neurosurgery. September 2024.
29. Mahmood F. Al-Zaidy MD, Mustafa Ismail MD, Ayaat F. Alasady MD, Mohammed S. Al-Hilfi MD , Mohammed S. Al-Sandooq MD, Fatimah Ayad MD, Mohamed Emara MD , Awfa Aktham Abdulateef MD, Samer S. Hoz MD. Suprasellar dermoid cyst masquerading as tumor: A case report. Asian Journal of Oncology. October 2024.
30. Maliya Delawan, Ahmed Muthana, Ali A. Dolachee, Muhammad Kashif, Abdullah M. Al-Qudah, Fatimah Oday Ahmed, Mohammed A. Alrawi, Samer S. Hoz. Microsurgery of Cerebral Arteriovenous Malformations in a Resource-Limited Setting: The First Case-Series from Iraq. World Neurosurgery. October 2024.
31. Ismail, Mustafa, Noor A. Hummadi, Noor K. Al-Waely, Saja A. Albanaa, Ali M. Neamah, Aktham O. Al-Khafaji, Sajjad Ghanim Al-Badri, Ahmed M. Jawad, and Samer S. Hoz. "Anterior communicating artery aneurysm microsurgery resulted in a proximal pseudoaneurysm." Adesh University Journal of Medical Sciences & Research 5, no. 2 (2024): 84-87.
32. Emara, Mohamed R., Alkawthar M. Abdulsada, Abdulaziz S. Alayyaf, Hussein A. Baban, Hala A. Al-Hchaimi, Mustafa Ismail, and Samer S. Hoz. "Ambient wing cistern: History, anatomy, imaging and approaches: An overview." World Neurosurgery: X (2024): 100395.
33. Samer S. Hoz, Li Ma, Ahmed Muthana, Mahmood Falah Al-Zaidy, Fatimah Oday Ahmed, Mustafa Ismail, Rachel C. Jacobs, Prateek Agarwal, Alhamza R. Al-Bayati, Raul G. Nogueira, Michael J. Lang, Bradley A. Gross1. Cranial nerve palsies and intracranial aneurysms: A

narrative review of patterns and outcomes. Surgical Neurology International. 09-Aug-2024;15:277.

34. Samer S. Hoz, Paolo Palmisciano, Mustafa Ismail, Ahmed Muthana, Edward J. Doyle, Mark D. Johnson, Jonathan A. Forbes, Charles J. Prestigiacomo, Ravi Samy, Mario Zuccarello1, Norberto Andaluz1. Minimally invasive presigmoid retrolabyrinthine suprameatal approach (PRSA): A cadaveric study for accessing premeatal anterior inferior cerebellar artery (AICA) aneurysms. Surgical Neurology International. 04-Oct-2024;15:364.
35. Samer S. Hoz, Paolo Palmisciano, Mustafa Ismail, Ahmed Muthana, Edward J. Doyle, Mark D. Johnson, Jonathan A. Forbes, Charles J. Prestigiacomo, Ravi Samy, Mario Zuccarello, Norberto Andaluz. Minimally invasive presigmoid retrolabyrinthine suprameatal approach (PRSA): A cadaveric study for accessing premeatal anterior inferior cerebellar artery (AICA) aneurysms. 04-Oct-2024;15:364
36. Alaraji ZA, Al-Ageely TA, Alaraji ZA, Abdulrazaq H, Atallah O, Ismail M, Samer S. Hoz. Neurosurgery-centred multidisciplinary team-based decisions: Experience from Iraq. Romanian Neurosurgery. 2023 Dec 15:430-2.
37. Khoailed AA, Abdulsada AM, Al-Hchaimi HA, Al-Khazaali YM, Aynona AM, Etaiwi AK, Ismail M, Samer S. Hoz. Temporary clipping in intracranial aneurysm surgery: History and development. Romanian Neurosurgery. 2023 Dec 15:433-7.
38. Al-Ageely TA, Ismail M, Al-Araji ZA, Abdulsada AM, Algburi HA, Akar NM, Samer S. Hoz. Effectiveness of Mentorships and Early Exposure in Neurosurgery. World Neurosurgery. 2023 Oct 1;178:e773-6.
39. Al-Ageely TA, Abdulhaleem A, Mohammed SA, Ismail M, Algburi H, Salih H, Samer S. Hoz. The central sulcus: Perioperative identification and surgical implication. Romanian Neurosurgery. 2023 Sep 15:272-7.
40. Ismail M, Hummadi N, Al-Waely N, Hadi R, Albanaa S, Daily S, Shamkhi M, Samer S. Hoz. 'Peacock tail'Clipping Technique for a Giant Middle Cerebral Artery Aneurysm: A Technical Note. Al-Kindy College Medical Journal. 2023 Aug 30;19(2):229-32.
41. Atallah O, Ismail M, Al-Khafaji AO, Samer S. Hoz. The Enigma of the Impervious Nobel Prize for Neurosurgeons. Cureus. 2023 Aug 28;15(8).

42. Delawan M, Sharma M, Ismail M, Algabri MH, Abdalridha RH, Alawadi MN, Alayya AS, Alrawi MA, Andaluz N, Samer S. Hoz. Methods of hemostasis in cranial neurosurgery: an anatomy-based stepwise review. World Neurosurgery. 2023 Aug 14.
43. Rowndzy II, Rashid HS, Ismail M, Saleh SA, Shaker NM, Muthana A, Ahmed MM, Rahem NH, Samer S. Hoz. Penetrating thoracic spine injury causing haemothorax: A case report. Romanian Neurosurgery. 2023 Jun 15:155-8.
44. Ismail M, Al-Hadeethi BM, Moushib AI, Algburi HA, Al-Khafaji AO, Al-Jehani H, Samer S. Hoz. Delayed intraoperative rupture of clipped aneurysm during the awaking from anaesthesia. Romanian Neurosurgery. 2023 Jun 15:198-201.
45. Dolachee A, Algburi H, Alsaad S, Ismail M, Samer S. Hoz. Similarities and differences between two coincidently gravitational bullet cases: A case report from Iraq. Romanian Neurosurgery. 2023 Jun 15:185-9.
46. Al-Ageely TA, Ismail M, Alsaadi SB, Salim FF, Kareem ZM, Talib SH, Jaafer H, Samer S. Hoz. Management of brain aneurysm neck-avulsion during clipping surgery: Illustrative case and literature review. Romanian Neurosurgery. 2023 Jun 15:164-9.
47. Ismail M, Al-Shalaji AK, Abdalnaby BS, Al-Khafaji AO, Kadhim AA, Al-Shakarchy RA, Zangana SA, Al-Rubaye AA, Samer S. Hoz. A giant A4-A5 distal anterior cerebral artery aneurysm treated with microsurgical clip reconstruction. Romanian Neurosurgery. 2023 Jun 15:218-23.
48. Al-Youzbaki RA, Mahmoud EH, Alsubaihawi ZA, Almeran MA, Albanaa SA, Samer S. Hoz. Incomplete Currarino triad in an adult woman: A case report. Romanian Neurosurgery. 2023 Mar 16:111-4.
49. Saheb AH, Al-Taie RH, Farooq IA, Taha AM, Naser HS, Yaseen ZM, Ismail M, Samer S. Hoz. Conservative management of intraventricular migrating intracranial bullet: A case report. Romanian Neurosurgery. 2023 Mar 15:59-63.
50. Talib SH, Sharma M, Ramanathan VP, Alfawares Y, Almufadhal MH, Ismail M, Samer S. Hoz. Spontaneous complete resolution of a giant cavernous carotid aneurysm in the setting of ipsilateral ICA occlusion. Romanian Neurosurgery. 2023 Mar 15:101-6.
51. Mohammad SA, Albulaihed SA, Ismail M, Alshuqayfi KM, Farooq IA, Al-Ageely TA, Palmisciano P, Andaluz N, Samer S. Hoz. Endolymphatic sac: A surreptitious anatomy for neurosurgeons. Surgical Neurology International. 2023;14(42):1.

52. Ismail M, Algburi HA, Al-Khazaal YM, Daily SK, Mohsin HE, Jaafar H, AbdulWahid J, Andaluz N, Samer S. Hoz. Academic productivity of Iraqi medical students in the field of neurosurgery: A literature review. Surgical Neurology International. 2023;14(52):1.
53. Etaiwi AM, Ismail M, Al-Ageely TA, Alasady AF, Jabbar AO, AbdulWahid J, Al-Zaidy MF, Samer S. Hoz. Retrograde cranio-orbital penetrating injury: A case report. Surgical Neurology International. 2023;14(11):1.
54. Ismail M, Algburi HA, Al-Khazaal YM, Daily SK, Mohsin HE, Jaafar H, AbdulWahid J, Andaluz N, Samer S. Hoz. Academic productivity of Iraqi medical students in the field of neurosurgery: A literature review. Surgical Neurology International. 2023;14(52):1.
55. Daily SK, Ismail M, Abdulmajeed AA, Aynona AM, Delawan M, Algabri MH, Samer S. Hoz. A case series of gyrus rectus arteriovenous malformation: Clinical characteristics, angioarchitecture, microsurgical treatment, and outcome. Surgical Neurology International. 2023;14(219):1.
56. Atallah O, Ismail M, Al-Khafaji A O, Samer S. Hoz. (August 28, 2023) The Enigma of the Impervious Nobel Prize for Neurosurgeons. Cureus 15(8): e44246.
57. Almurayati, M.E., Albanaa, S.A., Alsaadi, S.B., Al-Khafaji, A.O., Neamah, A.M., Hadi, R.T., Ismail, M. and Samer S. Hoz. 2023. Neurosurgery-Cases and Reviews.
58. Al-Ani SO, Albanaa SA, Alhajjaj EK, Al-Khafaji AO, Muhsen B, Samer S. Hoz. A Low-Velocity Semi-Wadcutter Bullet Resulting in a Fatal Traumatic Brain Injury: A Case Report. J Surg. 2023;8:1935.
59. Alrawi MA, Abdulqader MN, Salih HR, Saleh SA, Al-Ghuraibawi MA, Altaweel MM, Ismail M, Samer S. Hoz. Bilateral basal ganglia hemorrhage in a 2-year-old child. Surgical Neurology International. 2023;14.
60. Muthana A, Alsubaihawi ZA, Dolachee AA, Almurayati ME, Atallah O, Ismail M, Samer S. Hoz. Microsurgery for Grade III Cerebral Arteriovenous Malformations Related to the Eloquent Peri-Rolandic Territory: Case Series. Neurosurgery-Cases and Reviews. 2023.
61. Muthana A, Al-Gertani MR, Ahmed FO, Etaiwi AK, Al-Badri SG, Atallah O, Algabri MH, Ismail M, Samer S. Hoz. Occipital artery: Anatomical variations and neurosurgical applications. Surgical Neurology International. 2023;14.

62. Kareem ZM, Muthana A, Hassan SF, Ahmed FO, Hadi RT, Algburi HA, Atallah O, Ismail M, Samer S. Hoz. Supraorbital artery: Anatomical variations and neurosurgical applications. Surgical Neurology International. 2023;14.
63. Msebawy AS, Al-Araji ZA, Nazar A, Alayyaf A, Saleh SA, Merie SM, Alrawi MA, Ismail M, Samer S. Hoz. Surgical resection of pericallosal tuberculoma through contralateral approach: A case report. Surgical Neurology International. 2023;14.
64. Al-baidar RA, Ismail M, Elamin O, Ahmed MK, Abdulsada AM, Neamah AM, Al-Khafaji AO, Samer S. Hoz. Tangential gunshot wound to the head: A case report with review of literature. Romanian Neurosurgery. 2022 Dec 15:470-5.
65. Ismail M, Alsaadi SB, Badr MM, Al-Dhahi M, Abdulameer AO, Abdulsada AM, Al-Khafaji AO, Samer S. Hoz. Mobilization of the temporal pole as integrated step in microsurgical clipping of pure posteriorly directed posterior communicating artery aneurysm. Romanian Neurosurgery. 2022 Dec 15:476-8.
66. Abdulsada AM, Kareem ZM, Salih HA, Algburi HA, Ismail M, Samer S. Hoz. Deep motor cortex cavernoma resection supported by navigational intraoperative monitoring: A case report. Romanian Neurosurgery. 2022 Dec 15:465-9.
67. Al-Smaysim AM, Alhayali WK, Alsaadi SB, Abdulameer AO, Ismail M, Samer S. Hoz. Endoscopic third ventriculostomy: Complications and avoidance. Romanian Neurosurgery. 2022 Dec 15:479-82.
68. Ismail M, Alshalchi AK, Badr MM, Abdulameer AO, Algburi HA, Al-Taie RH, Al-Lami S, Al-Khafaji AO, Samer S. Hoz. Impact of dome projection on operative steps during clipping of a ruptured pure posteriorly directed posterior communicating artery aneurysms. Romanian Neurosurgery. 2022 Sep 15:355-8.
69. Ismail M, Talib SH, Albairmani S, Al-Khafaji AO, Al-Jehani H, Samer S. Hoz. Coil migration during pressure-cooker technique for cerebral AVM: A case report. Romanian Neurosurgery. 2022 Sep 15:350-4.
70. Ismail M, Abdulqader MN, Ahmed FO, Al-Khafaji AO, Al-Jehani H, Samer S. Hoz. Cervical carotid artery vasospasm during cerebral angiography. Romanian Neurosurgery. 2022 Sep 15:346-9.

71. Palmisciano P, Ferini G, Watanabe G, Conching A, Ogasawara C, Scalia G, Bin-Alamer O, Haider AS, Passanisi M, Maugeri R, Samer S. Hoz. Surgical Management of Craniovertebral Junction Schwannomas: A Systematic Review. Current Oncology. 2022 Jul 9;29(7):4842-55.
72. khashea Mustafa M, Matti WE, Kadhum H, Kareem ZM, Alsubaihawi ZA, Al-Sharshahi ZF, Samer S. Hoz. Giant cerebral hydatid cyst manifesting as seizures in a child: A case report and literature review. Indonesian Journal of Neurosurgery. 2022 Jun 4;5(2):51-5.
73. Al-Sharshahi ZF, Alsubaihawi ZA, Kareem ZM, Ali N, Albanaa SA, Al-Khafaji AO, Neamah AM, Samer S. Hoz. Adult primary frontal ganglioneuroma: A case report. Indonesian Journal of Neurosurgery. 2022 Jun 4;5(2):48-50.
74. Ranjha KU, Farooq M, Samer S. Hoz. Commentary: Altmetrics Versus Bibliometrics in Neurosurgery—Finding a Balance. Neurosurgery. 2022 May 17:10-227.
75. Ismail M, Al-Ageely TA, Talib SH, Hadi RT, Al-Taie RH, Aktham AA, Alrawi MA, Salih HR, Al-Jehani H, Samer S. Hoz. Atypical slow-flow paramedian AVM with venous varix. Surgical Neurology International. 2022;13.
76. Al-Ageely TA, Ismail M, Mohammed SA, Al-Delfi AH, Alshedidi MS, Al-Jaberi MB, Almufadhal MH, Abdulateef AA, Aljuboori Z, Al-Jehani H, Samer S. Hoz. Failure of tandem flow diversion for intracranial aneurysms: Literature review and illustrative case. Surgical Neurology International. 2022;13.
77. Ismail M, Al-Ageely TA, Alzerkani MA, Al-Khazaali YM, Salih HA, Al-Khafaji AO, Kareem ZM, Abdulsada AM, Salih HR, Samer S. Hoz. Extracranial carotid localized fibromuscular dysplasia: A case report and literature review. Surgical Neurology International. 2022;13.
78. Salih HR, Jaafer H, Ismail M, Khallaf AK, Mohammed AJ, Al-Mosawy MS, Naser HS, Maulood ZT, Hafedh AN, Samer S. Hoz. Extensive tension pneumocephalus presented in the setting of a challenging etiology. Surgical Neurology International. 2022;13.
79. Algburi HA, Sharma M, Ismail M, Albulaihed SA, Al-Gertani MR, Majeed SN, Hasan HM, Idris OS, Andaluz N, Samer S. Hoz. The coexistence of anterior communicating artery aneurysm and meningioma: A literature review and illustrative case. Surgical Neurology International. 2022;13.
80. Al-Alousi HM, Al-Kubaisi KT, Ismail M, Al-Ageely TA, Abdulameer AO, Aluaibi SA, Al-Taie RH, Samer S. Hoz. Transbasal penetrating traumatic brain injury caused by a rifle rod: A case report. Surgical Neurology International. 2022;13.

81. AbdulWahid J, Ismail M, Al-Mosawy MS, Abdulsada AM, Al-Ageely TA, Samer S. Hoz. Ins and outs in deciding a future career in neurosurgery: A medical student's perspective. Surgical Neurology International. 2022;13.

82. Abdulqader MN, Ismail M, Al-Khafaji AO, Al-Ageely TA, Kareem ZM, Al-Baider RA, Albairmani SS, Ayad F, Samer S. Hoz. Brown-Sequard syndrome associated with a spinal cord injury caused by a retained screwdriver: A case report and literature review. Surgical Neurology International. 2022;13.

83. Yousif RS, Omar AM, Ismail M, Hamouda WO, Alkhafaji AO, Samer S. Hoz. Excellent recovery after nonmissile penetrating traumatic brain injury in a child: A case report. Surgical Neurology International. 2022;13.

84. Maher Khashea Mustafa, Wamedh E. Matti, Hussain J. Kadhum, Zahraa M. Kareem, Zahraa A. Alsubaihawi, Zahraa F. Al-Sharshahi, Samer S. Hoz. Giant cerebral hydatid cyst manifesting as seizures in a child: A case report and literature review. Indonesian Journal of Neurosurgery. 6, 2022.

85. Zahraa F. Alsharshahi, Zahraa A. Alsubaihawi, Zahraa M. Kareem, Narges Ali, Saja A. Albanaa, Aktham O. Al-Khafaji, Ali M. Neamah, Samer S. Hoz. Adult primary frontal ganglioneuroma: A case report. Indonesian Journal of Neurosurgery. 6, 2022.

86. Sadiqo R, Abdulsada AM, Ismail M, Samer S. Hoz. Ectopic schwannoma of the sellar region in a 1-year-old child: A case report and review of literature. Surgical Neurology International. 2022;13.

87. Mustafa MK, Matti WE, Kadhum HJ, Alsubaihawi ZA, Kareem ZM, Al-Sharshahi ZF, Samer S. Hoz. Spontaneous intracerebral haemorrhage as an initial presentation of a choriocarcinoma: A case report. Romanian Neurosurgery. 2021 Mar 9:48-51.

88. Hafedh AN, Aktham AA, Al-Sharshahi ZF, Al-Jorani AI, Albairamani S, Alsubaihawi ZA, Al-Khafaji AO, Samer S. Hoz. Primary multiple cerebral hydatid disease in a young patient with surgically-treated intracerebral haemorrhage: A case report. Romanian Neurosurgery. 2021 Mar 9:71-4.

89. Serra Sencer, Mohamed M. Arnaout, Hosam Al-Jehani M, Zahraa A. Alsubaihawi, Zahraa F. Al-Sharshahi, Samer S. Hoz. The Spectrum of Venous Anomalies Associated with Atretic Parietal Cephaloceles: A Literature Review. Surgical Neurology International. 2021.

90. Al-Sharshahi, Z. F., H. R. Salih, A. A. Aktham, M. A. Shamkhi, M. A. Murayati, N. F. Hassan, A. O. Al-Khafaji and Samer S. Hoz (2021). "Letter to the Editor: Cadaver-Free Simulation Training in Microneurosurgery: An Experience from Iraq." World Neurosurg 151: 310-312.
91. Al-Sharshahi Z, Al-Hemiery H, Albaqer H, Hamandi Y, Al-Awadi O, Samer S. Hoz. Following the footprints of pioneers on neurosurgery in Iraq: Abdul Hadi Al-Khalili. Surgical Neurology International. 2021;12:110.
92. Al-Sharshahi ZF, Albanaa SA, Jawad AM, Al-Waely NK, Hummadi NA, Samer S. Hoz. Dolichoectatic middle cerebral artery masquerading as cerebral cavernous malformation: A case report and review of literature. Romanian Neurosurgery. 2020 Dec 16:498-503.
93. Albanaa SA, Al-Sharshahi ZF, Hummadi NA, Al-Waely NK, Alshakarchy RA, Neamah AM, Alkhafaji AO, Samer S. Hoz. Enlarged anterior communicating artery masquerading as intracranial aneurysm: Case report. Romanian Neurosurgery. 2020 Sep 15:455-8.
94. Al-Smaysim AM, Alhayali WK, Lafta MH, Al-Sharshahi ZF, Abdulrazzaq AS, Jassam AK, Samer S. Hoz. A classification system for penetrating traumatic brain injuries caused by tear-gas canisters. World J Pharm Pharmaceut Sci. 2020 Feb 7;9(4):156-62.
95. Aktham A, AbdulAzeez MM, Samer S. Hoz. Surgical Intervention of Intracerebral Hematoma Caused by Ruptured Middle Cerebral Artery Aneurysm in Neurosurgery Teaching Hospital, Baghdad, Iraq. Neurology India. 2020;68(1):124-31.
96. Alsaadi SB, Mohammed SA, Kareem ZM, Almurayati M, Samer S. Hoz. Surgical control over superior sagittal sinus injury due to metallic ceiling fan-blade injury. Mustansiriya Medical Journal. 2020 Jan 1;19(1):34.
97. Al-Khafaji AO, Al-Sharshahi ZF, Lee RP, Alsubaihawi ZA, Dolachee AA, Samer S. Hoz. Unilateral absence of the internal carotid artery associated with anterior communicating artery aneurysms: Systematic review and a proposed management algorithm. Surg Neurol Int. 2020;11:221.
98. Abdelrazaq SS, Al Ramadan AH, Dolachee AA, AbdulAzeez MM, Abdulrazzaq AS, Rashid AS, Samer S. Hoz. Hydatid cyst of the quadrigeminal cistern: A case report for unusual location with literature review. Romanian Neurosurgery. 2019 Jun 15:150-5.
99. Moscote-Salazar LR, Dolachee AA, Narvaez–Rojas A, Al–Saadi HA, Najim AA, Abdulreda AK, Mahmood AO, Mohammed HJ, Samer S. Hoz. Preoperative embolization of skull–base tumors: Indications, utility, and concerns. Journal of Acute Disease. 2019 May 1;8(3):89.

100. Lafta G, Dolachee A, Al-Zubaidi A, Samer S. Hoz. A death calls from unsafe heights. a study of factors influencing the outcome of surgically treated pediatric head trauma patients in baghdad. International Journal of Research in Pharmaceutical Sciences. 2019;10:1997-2001.

101. Dolachee A, Lafta G, Al-Zubaidi A, Samer S. Hoz. Rules of rhoton and saccular intracranial aneurysms: an in vivo radiological-anatomical confirmatory study in iraqi population. Annals of Tropical Medicine and Public Health. 2019;22.

102. AbdulAzeez MM, Dolachee AA, Huber PZ, Romario MF, Obaid HA, Arakwazi AH, Altaweel MM, Samer S. Hoz. Intracranial ricocheted-bullet injuries: An overview and illustrative case. Journal of Acute Disease. 2018 Sep 1;7(5):186.

103. Alhillo HT, Sadik HA, Gheni TN, Samer S. Hoz. Rare occurrence of a huge traumatic extradural haematoma in a patient with an ipsilateral sylvian arachnoid cyst. BMJ case reports. 2018;11(1).

104. Alhillo HT, Arnaout MM, Radhi HS, Al-Dhahir MA, Moscote-Salazar LR, Samer S. Hoz. Direct head injury caused by a tear gas cartridge. Questions on safety: A case report from Iraq and review of the literature. J Clin Neurosci. 2018;56:179-82.

105. AbdulAzeez M, Huber P-Z, Alsaadi S, Vladimir C-N, Salazar L, Samer S. Hoz. Cranio-cervical bone hyperpneumatization: An overview and illustrative case. Journal of Acute Disease. 2018;7(4):145-8.

Books

1. Book: Samer S. Hoz: Vascular neurosurgery: In multiple-choice questions. 1st 03/2017; Springer International Publishing., ISBN: 978-3-319-49187-5, DOI:10.1007/978-3-319-49187-5.
2. Book: Samer S. Hoz, Cherian I, Dolachee A, Zahraa F. Al-Sharshahi, Salih H, AlRawi M et al. Neurotrauma - In Multiple-Choice Questions, 1st ed. Springer; 2021. ISBN 978-3-030-80868-6.
3. Book: Samer S. Hoz, Dolachee, A.A., Salih, H.R., Aljuboori, Z.S., Selbi, W.D., Al-Dayri, G., Al-Salihi, M.M.: Pineal neurosurgery. 1st 10/2020; Springer International Publishing., ISBN: 978-3-030-53190-4, DOI: 10.1007/978-3-030-53191-1.
4. Book: Salih HR, Samer S. Hoz, Dolachee AA, Alrawi MA, Aljuboori Z, Sharma M, Ismail M, Andaluz N. Cerebral Ventricles - In Multiple-Choice Questions, 1st ed. Springer; November 2023. ISBN 978-3-031-42341-3.
5. Book: Samer S. Hoz, Zahraa F. Al-Sharshahi., Ghanim Teeba, M., et al. Neurosurgery Board Favorites: Crossword Puzzles. 1st ed. IngramSpark; 2021. ISBN-13: 978-0-578-85444-1
6. Book: Salih HR, Samer S. Hoz, Dolachee AA, Alrawi MA, Aljuboori Z, Sharma M, Ismail M, Andaluz N. Cerebral Ventricles - In Multiple-Choice Questions, 1st ed. Springer; November 2023. ISBN 978-3-031-42341-3.
7. Book: Samer S. Hoz, Al Ramadan AH, Pople I., Mohammed N., Hamouda WO., El Damaty A., Mustafa Ismail M. Pediatric Neurosurgery- In Multiple-Choice Questions, 1st ed. Springer; March 2024. ISBN 978-3-031-49572-4.
8. Book: Samer S. Hoz, Oday Atallah, Li Ma, Zaid Aljuboori, Mayur Sharma, Mustafa Ismail, Maliya Delawan. Surgical Neuro-Oncology – In Multiple Choice Questions, 1 st ed. Springer; 16 April 2024. ISBN 978-3-031-53642-7.
9. Book: Samer Hoz, Asmaa H. AL-Sharee, Mustafa Ismail Ali A. Dolachee, Osman Elamin Oday Atallah, Maliya Delawan. Neuroradiology Board's Favorites 100 MRI-Based Pathology-Proven Cases Supplied with 170 MCQs. 1 st ed. Springer. October 2024. ISBN 978-3-031-64260-9.

10. Book: Samer S. Hoz, Ali M. Neamah, Ahmed Muthana, Abrar A. Khoailed, Maliya Delawan, Mohammed Al-Dhahir. Neuroanatomy Board Favorites Crossword Puzzles. HOZ NeuroSurgery LAB; 1st edition (July 8, 2024).

ɔu Should NEVER Walk Alone
z Neurosurgery Mentorship

gallery captures the essence of the Hoz Neurosurgery Mentorship, ɪwcasing moments of growth, learning, and transformation. From ɾating room experiences to hands-on training, global collaborations, mentees' achievements, these images tell the story of a mentorship shapes future neurosurgeons. Each photo represents a milestone in journey of mentorship, dedication, and excellence.

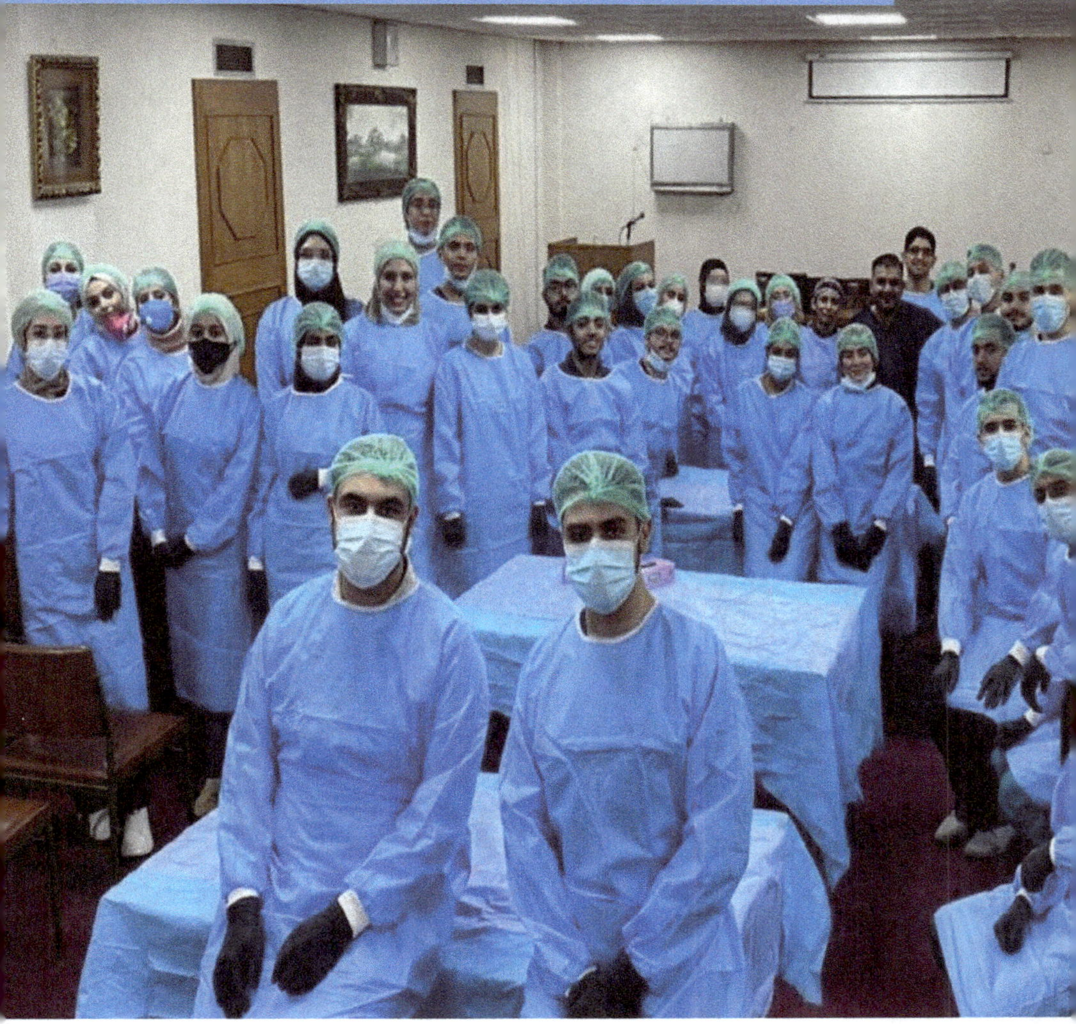

The Beginnings of the Mentorship

First Mentorship Meeting and Orientation Session
Date: May 15, 2021
Occasion: Inaugural meeting of the 2021 Mentorship Group
Location: First online Zoom session
This session marked the beginning of an inspiring journey, introducing mentees to the mentorship program's vision, goals, and expectations. It sets the foundation for meaningful learning, collaboration, and professional growth.

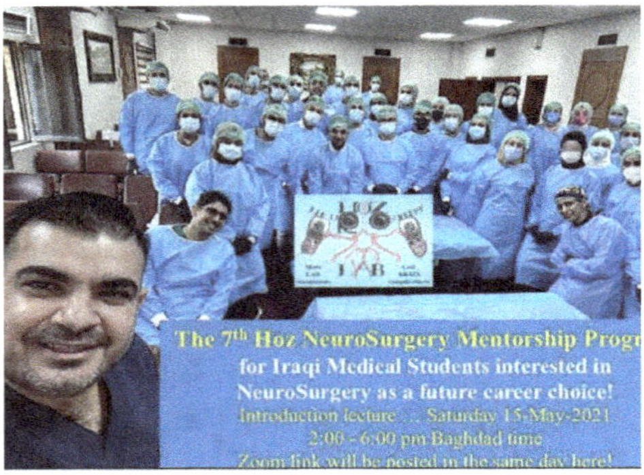
The 7th Hoz NeuroSurgery Mentorship Progr
for Iraqi Medical Students interested in
NeuroSurgery as a future career choice!
Introduction lecture … Saturday 15-May-2021
2:00 - 6:00 pm Baghdad time
Zoom link will be posted in the same day here!

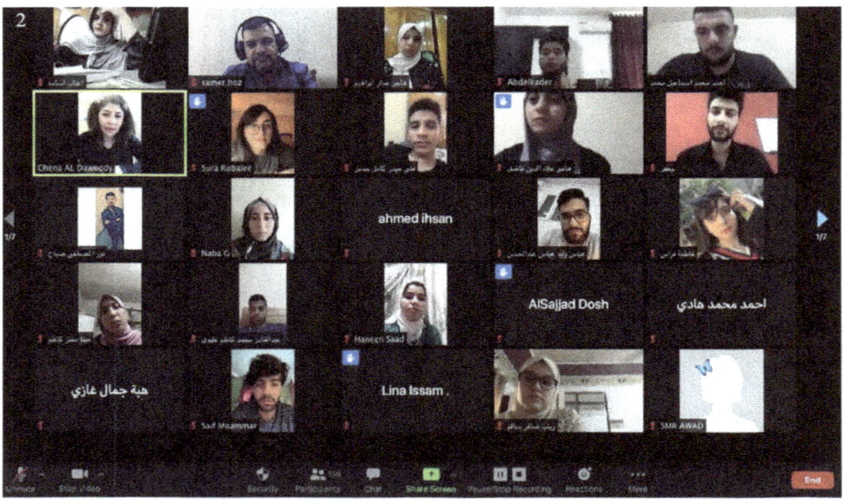
ahmed ihsan
AlSajjad Dosh
احمد محمد هادي
هبة جمال غازي
Lina Issam .

The Mentorship in Action

Date: January 4, 2022
Occasion: Mentees had the opportunity to observe a neurosurgical procedure and gain clinical exposure.
Location: Al-Moayad Private Hospital, Baghdad
This session provided mentees with a valuable firsthand experience in the operating room, enhancing their understanding of neurosurgical techniques and procedures.

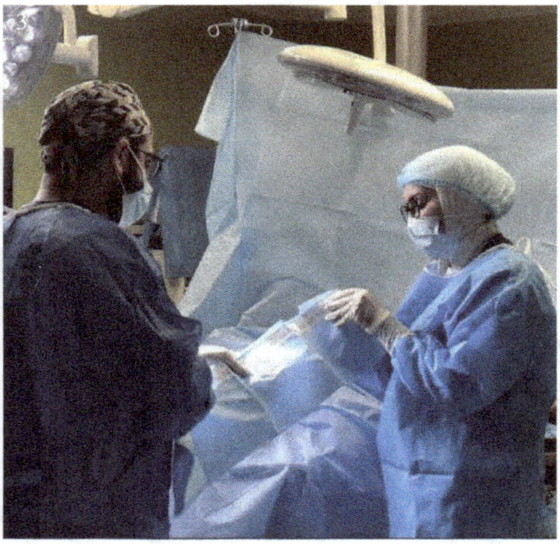

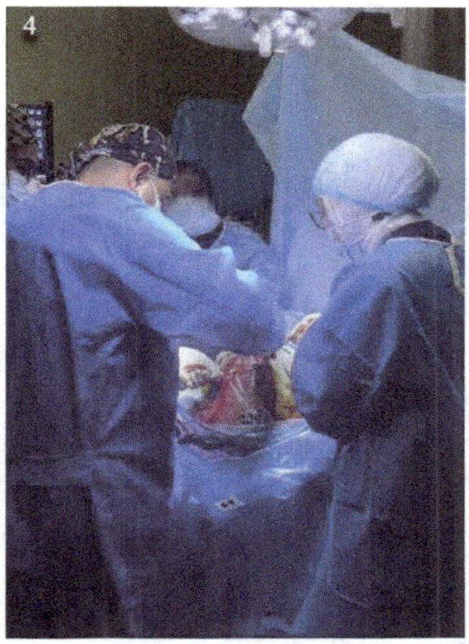

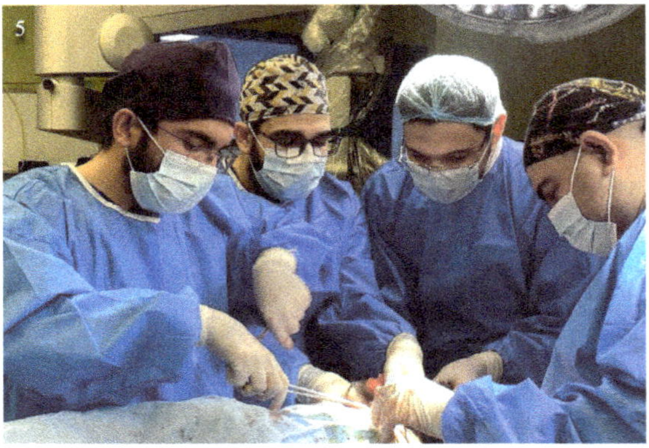

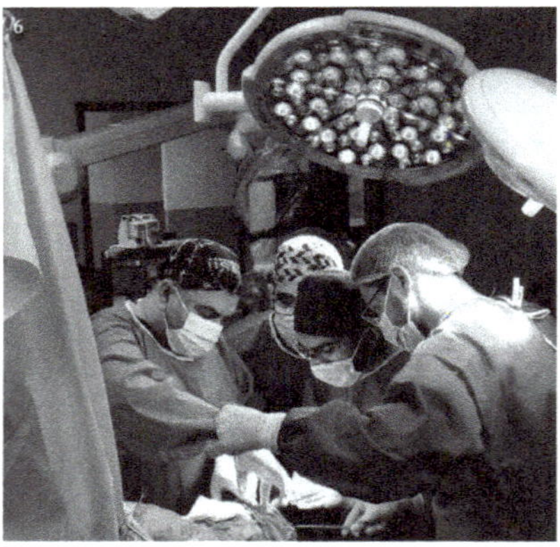

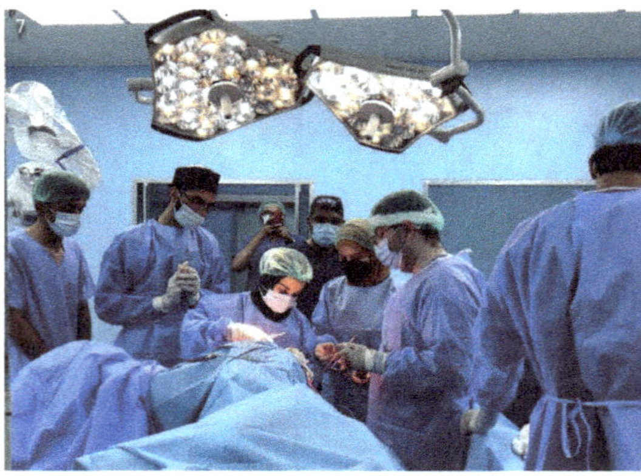

ate: June 2, 2021

ccasion: Mentees had the opportunity to observe a neurosurgical procedure and gain clinical exposure.

ocation: Neurosurgery Teaching Hospital, Baghdad

uring this session, the neurosurgeon provided step-by-step explanations of the procedure, guiding mentees rough the anatomical structures and surgical techniques being performed. This interactive learning experience lowed them to develop a deeper understanding of neurosurgical interventions.

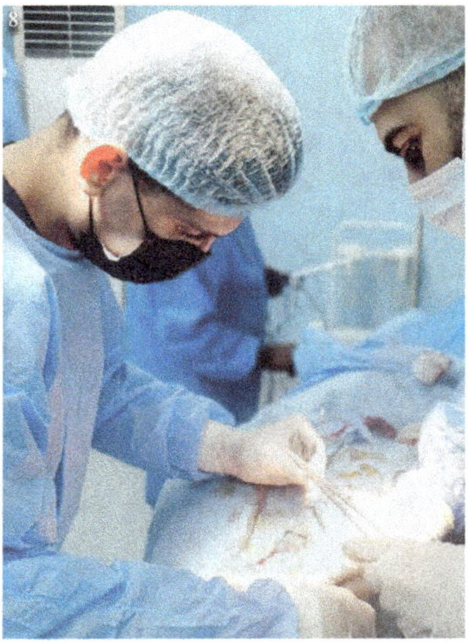

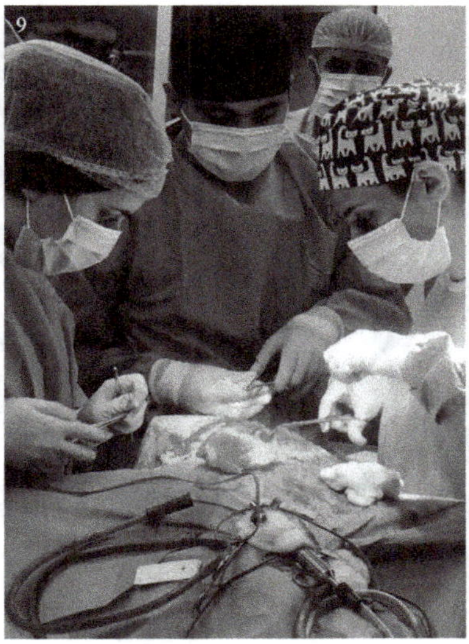

Date: June 10, 2021

Occasion: Mentees had the opportunity to observe a neurosurgical procedure and gain clinical expo:

Location: Neurosurgery Teaching Hospital, Baghdad

During this session, the neurosurgeon provided real-time explanations of each step of the procec highlighting key anatomical structures and surgical techniques. The observation experience allowed mer to enhance their understanding of neurosurgical workflows in a high-stakes clinical environment.

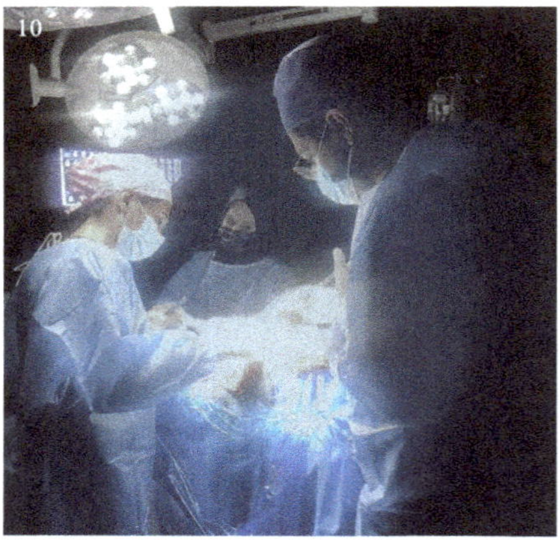

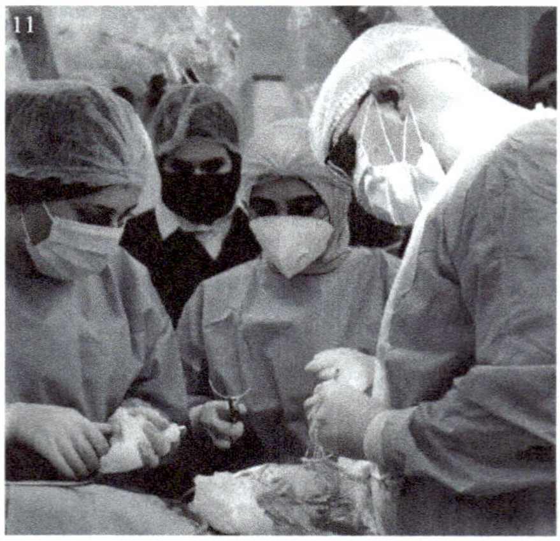

Date: June 15, 2021

Occasion: Mentees had the opportunity to observe a neurosurgical procedure and gain clinical exposure.

Location: Neurosurgery Teaching Hospital, Baghdad

In this session, mentees observed the surgery remotely via a live broadcast within the operating room. The neurosurgeon provided detailed explanations of the procedure, ensuring the mentees could follow each step while discussing key anatomical and surgical principles. This setup allowed for an interactive learning experience without disrupting the surgical workflow.

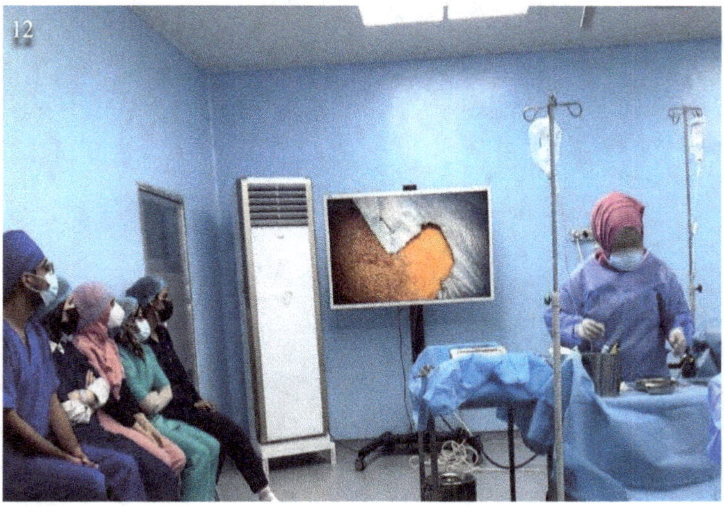

Date: June 20, 2021

Occasion: Mentees had the opportunity to engage in neurosurgical skill lab activities, practicing fundamental techniques and enhancing their hands-on experience.

Location: Neurosurgery Teaching Hospital, Baghdad

During this session, mentees were introduced to essential neurosurgical skills, including suturing techniques, handling microsurgical instruments, and precision training. Under expert supervision, they gained practical exposure to surgical principles, fostering their technical proficiency and confidence in neurosurgical procedures.

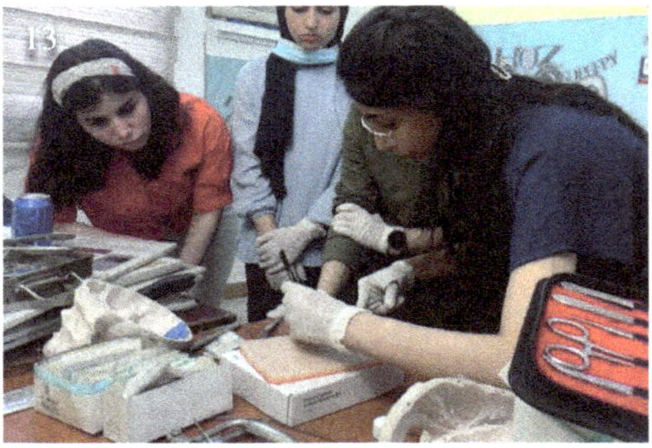

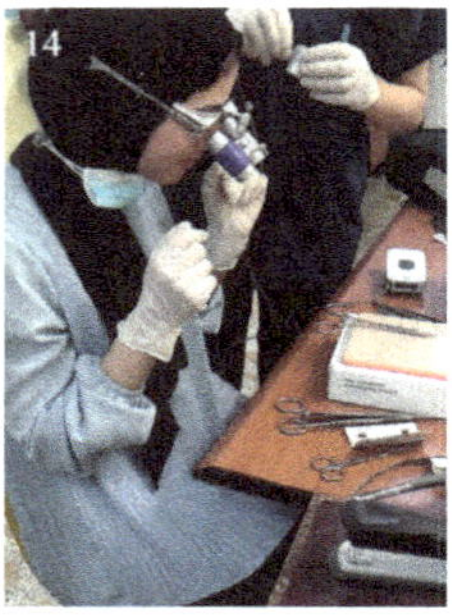

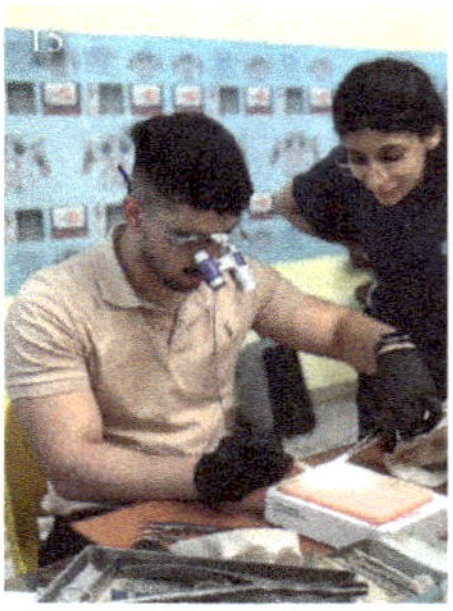

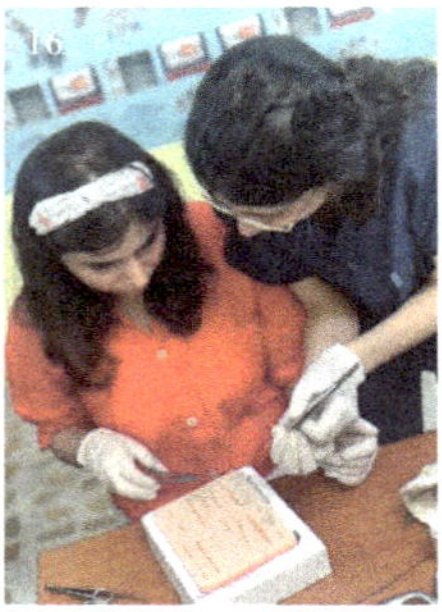

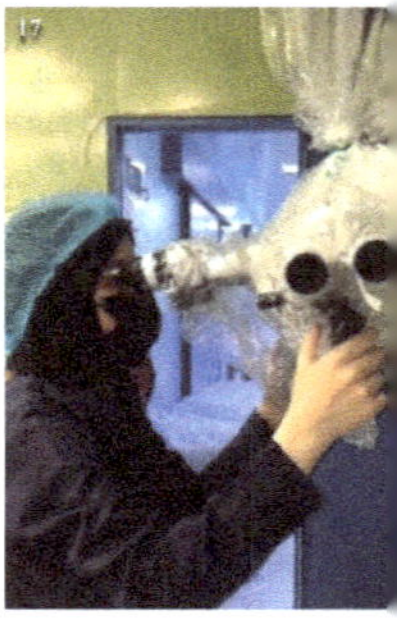

te: July 7, 2021

casion: Mentees had the opportunity to observe an endovascular neurosurgical procedure and gain clinical posure.

cation: Al-Moayad Private Hospital, Baghdad

ring this session, mentees observed a specialized endovascular neurosurgical procedure, gaining insights o minimally invasive techniques used to treat vascular conditions. The neurosurgeon provided detailed planations of catheter navigation, fluoroscopic imaging, and interventional techniques, enhancing the ntees' understanding of endovascular approaches in neurosurgery.

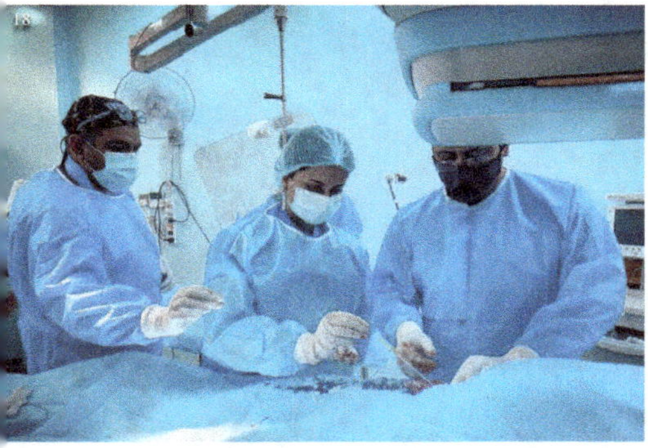

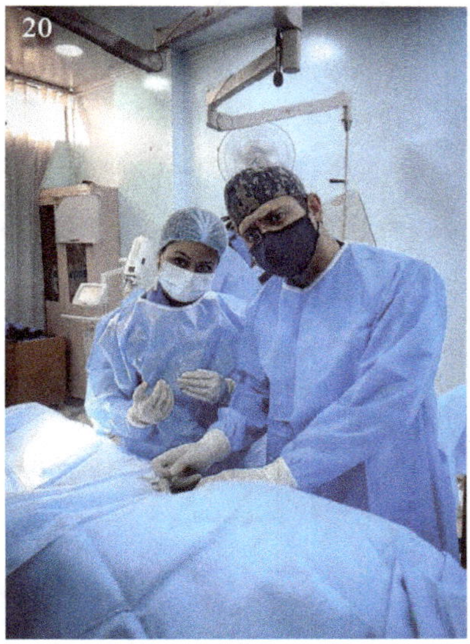

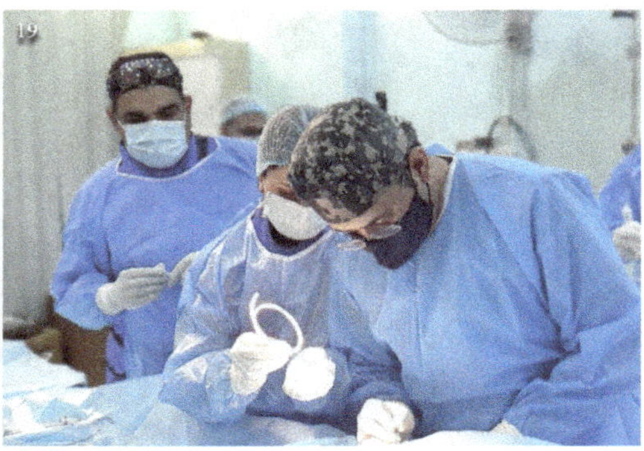

Date: August 17, 2021

Occasion: Mentees had the opportunity to observe a neurosurgical procedure and gain hands-on experience in using a surgical microscope.

Location: Neurosurgery Teaching Hospital, Baghdad

During this session, mentees were introduced to the fundamentals of microsurgery, including microscope navigation, fine motor control, and high-precision techniques. Under expert supervision, they practiced handling the microscope, enhancing their understanding of magnification-based surgical approaches in neurosurgery.

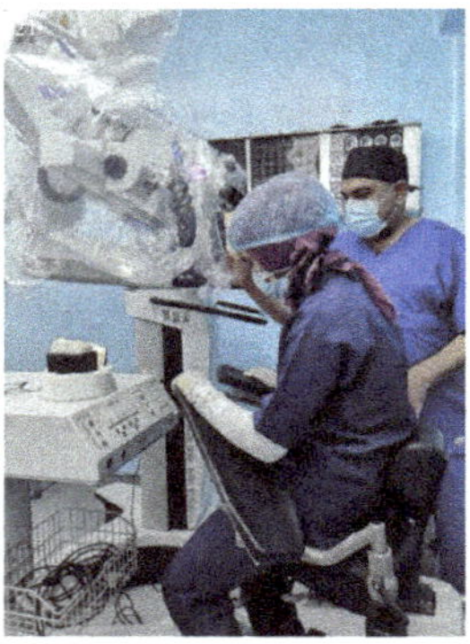

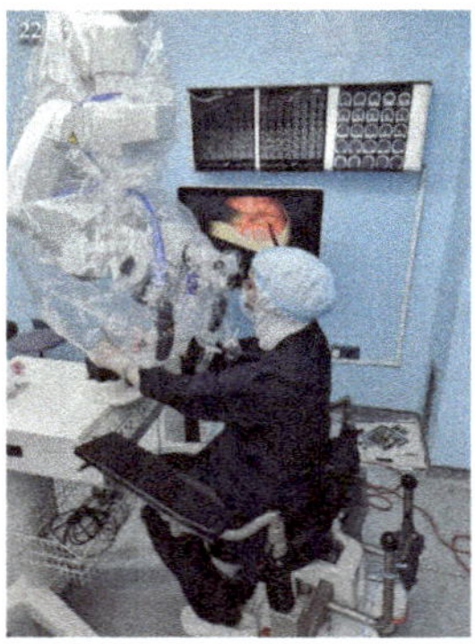

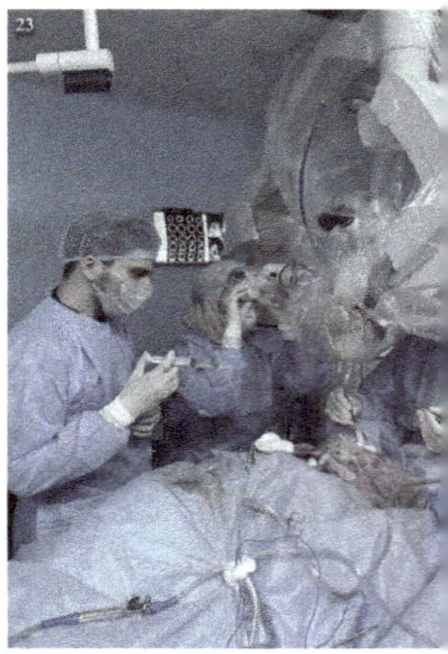

Date: October 5, 2021

Occasion: Mentees had the opportunity to observe a neurosurgical procedure and gain clinical exposure.

Location: Neurosurgery Teaching Hospital, Baghdad

This session offered mentees an in-depth look into the surgical management of neurological conditions. The neurosurgeon guided them through the procedure, explaining decision-making processes, intraoperative challenges, and key neurosurgical principles, providing a valuable learning experience in a high-stakes environment.

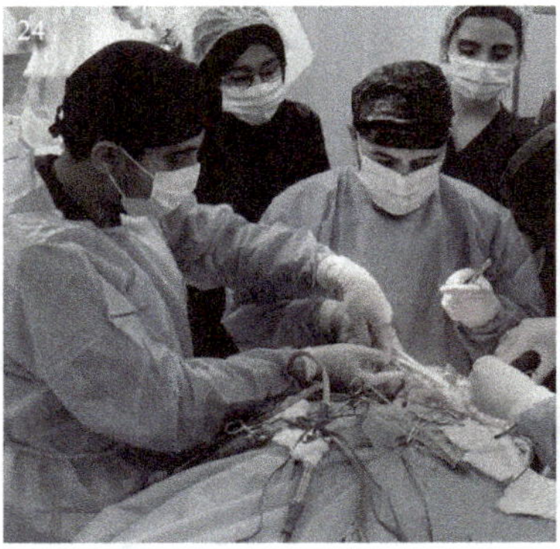

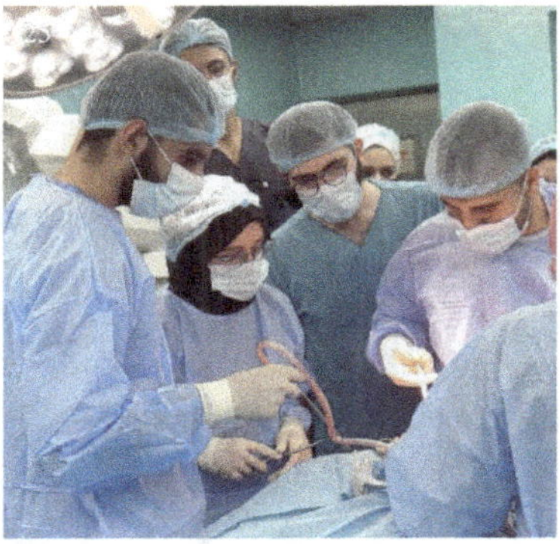

26
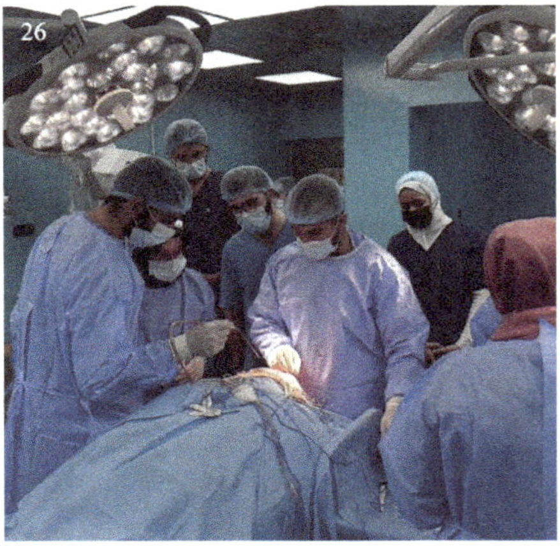

27
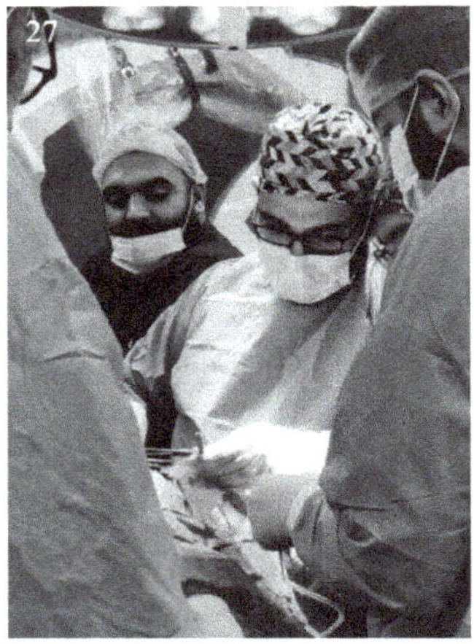

28
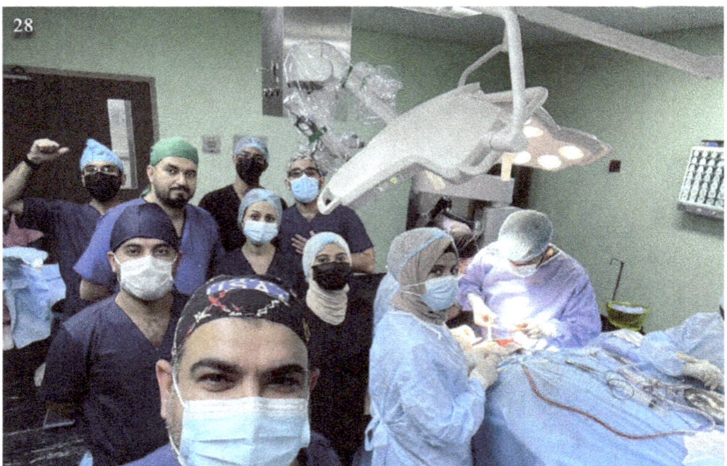

Date: December 20, 2021

Occasion: Mentees had the opportunity to observe an endovascular neurosurgical procedure and gain clinical exposure.

Location: Al-Moayad Private Hospital, Baghdad

During this session, mentees observed a minimally invasive endovascular procedure, learning about catheter-based interventions for neurovascular conditions. The neurosurgeon provided detailed explanations of fluoroscopic imaging, vascular navigation, and interventional techniques, enhancing their understanding of endovascular neurosurgery.

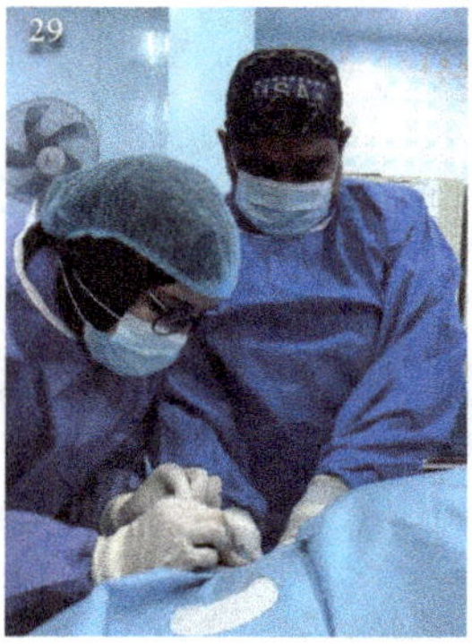

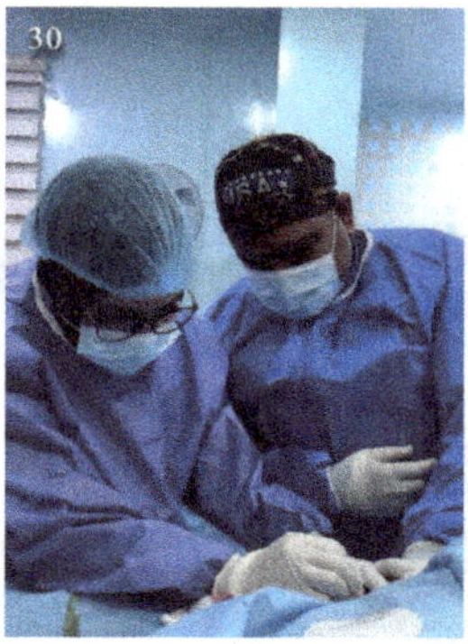

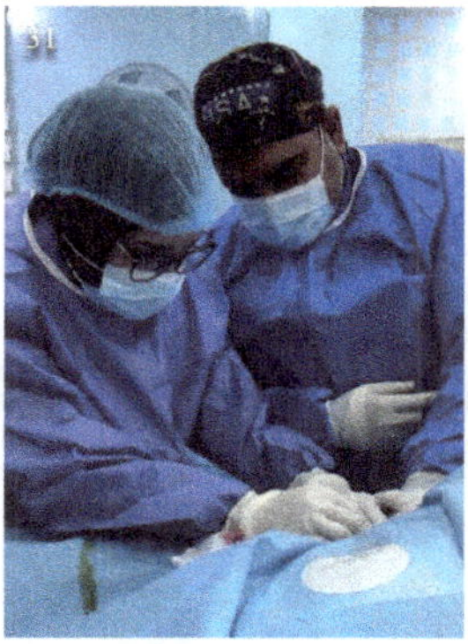

Date: December 20, 2021

Occasion: Mentees had the opportunity to observe a cranial neurosurgical procedure, focusing on the intricacies of dura mater dissection and hemostatic techniques.

Location: Al-Moayad Private Hospital, Baghdad

During this session, mentees observed a cranial surgery, where the neurosurgeon demonstrated step-by-step techniques, including precise scalpel handling, dural opening, and meticulous hemostasis using bipolar coagulation. The neurosurgical team provided real-time explanations of key anatomical landmarks and intraoperative decision-making, allowing mentees to gain a comprehensive understanding of cranial surgical interventions.

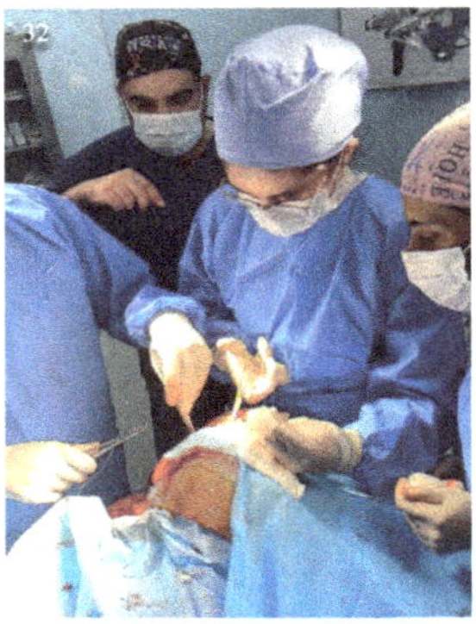

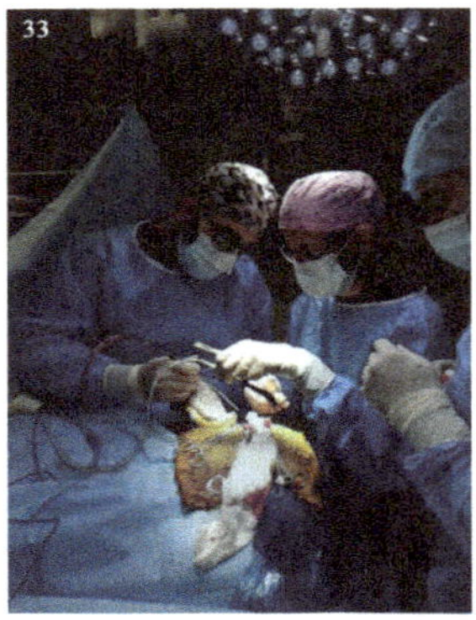

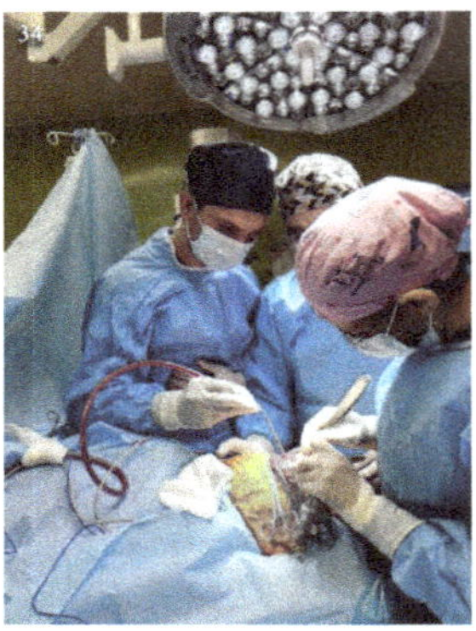

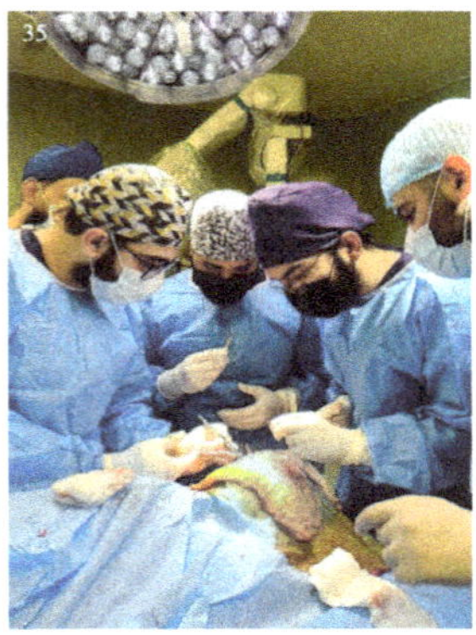

)ate: February 5, 2022

)ccasion: Mentees had the opportunity to observe a cranial neurosurgical procedure, focusing on skull flap levation and dural repair techniques.

.ocation: Al-Moayad Private Hospital, Baghdad

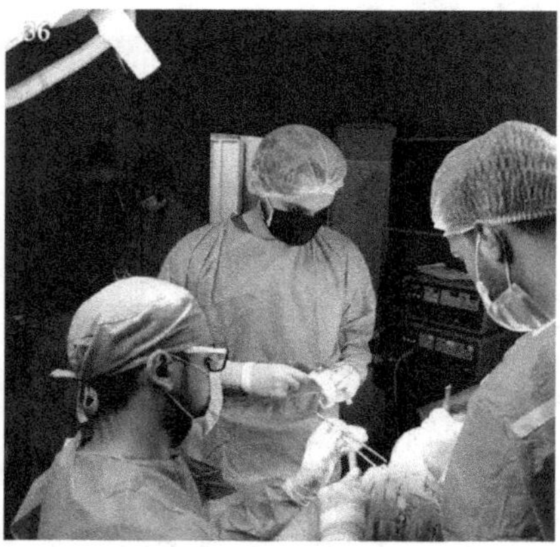

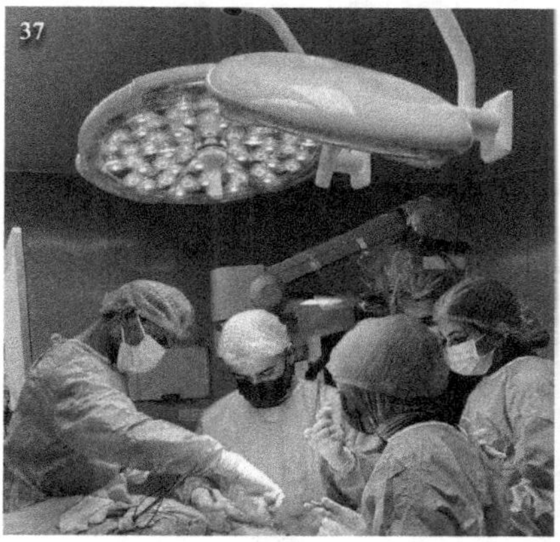

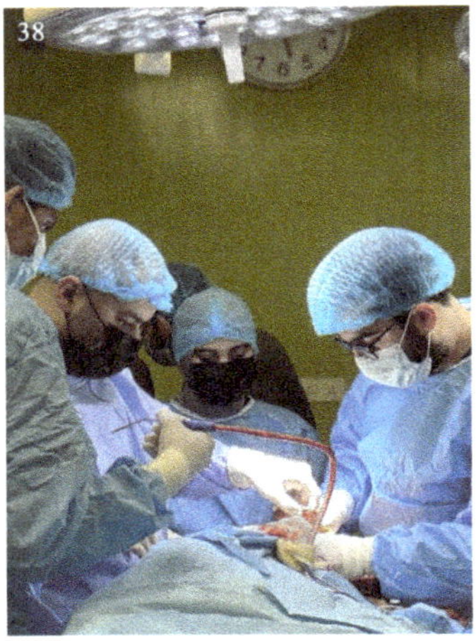

38

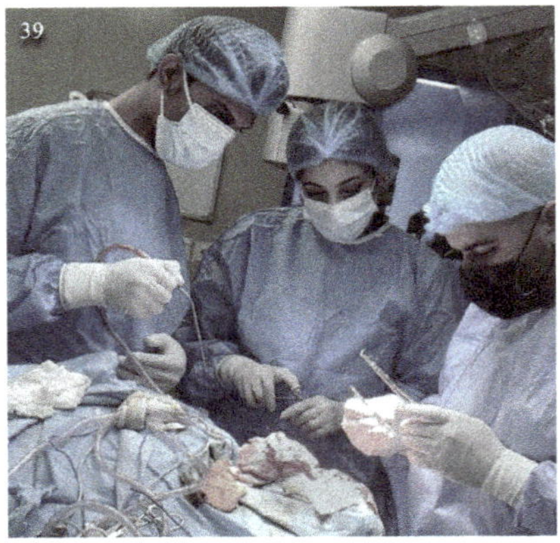

39

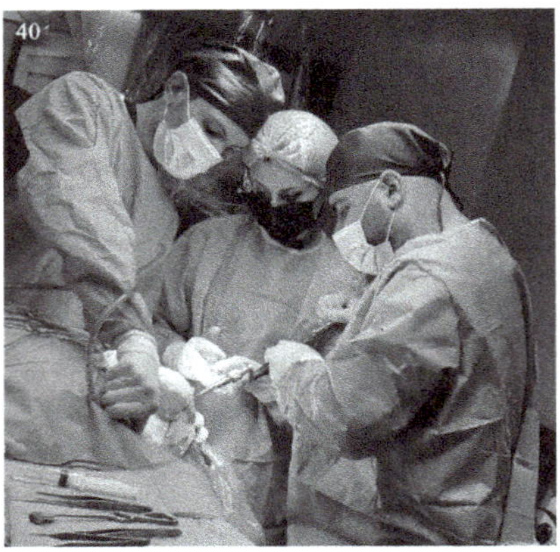

40

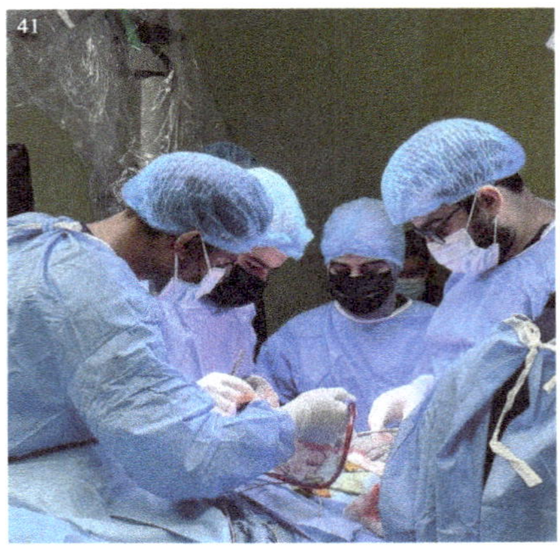

41

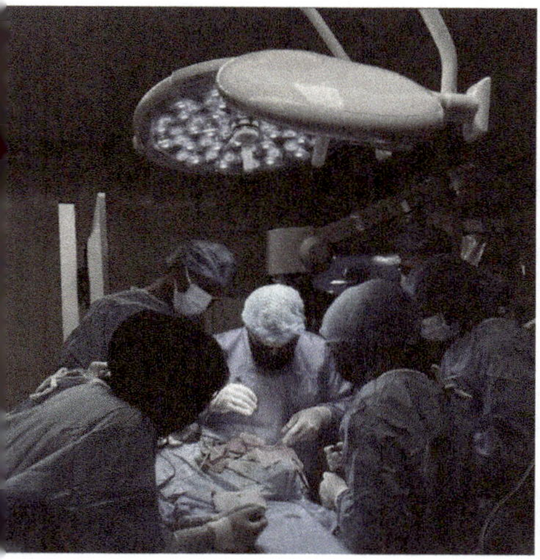

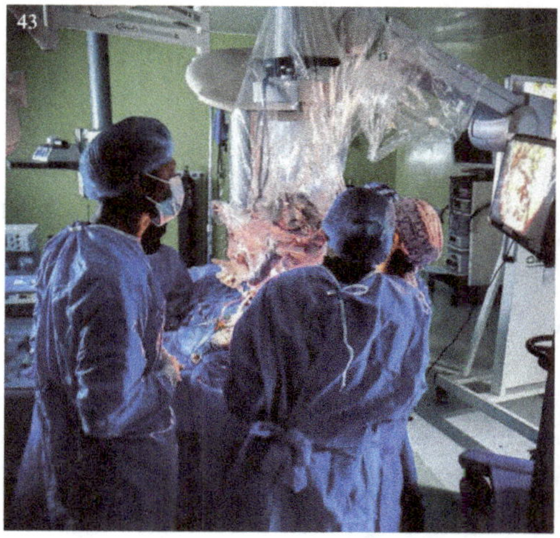

43

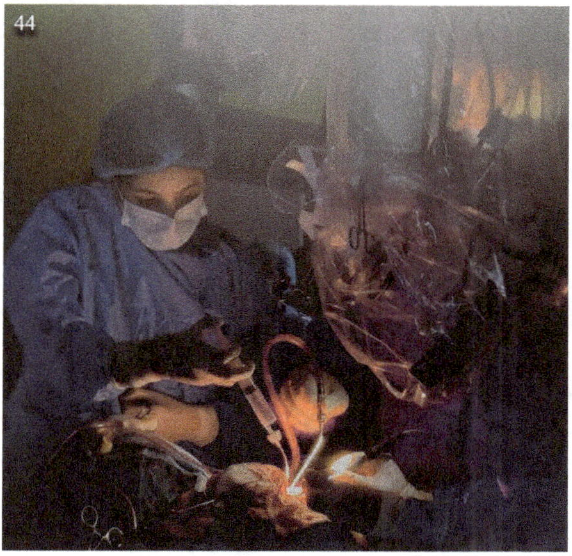

44

Date: February 5, 2022

Occasion: Mentees had the opportunity to observe an endovascular neurosurgical procedure, focusing on catheter-based interventions and real-time fluoroscopic imaging.

Location: Al-Moayad Private Hospital, Baghdad

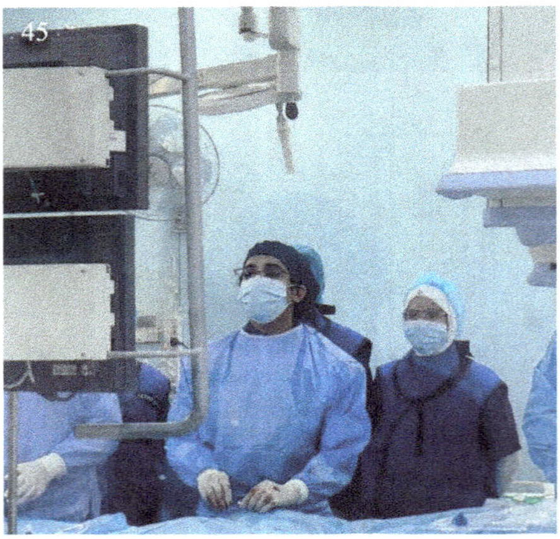

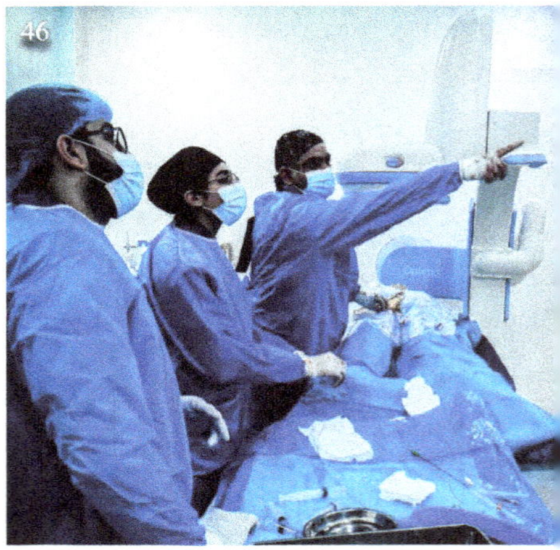

Date: February 7, 2022

Occasion: Mentees had the opportunity to observe a **cranial neurosurgical procedure**, focusing on microsurgical dissection and vascular control techniques.

Location: Al-Moayad Private Hospital, Baghdad

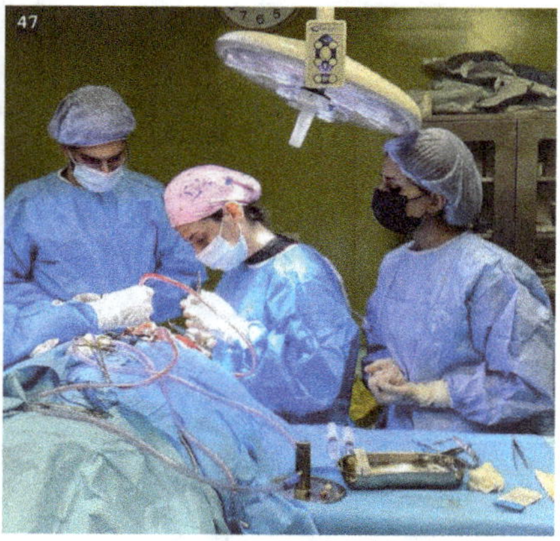

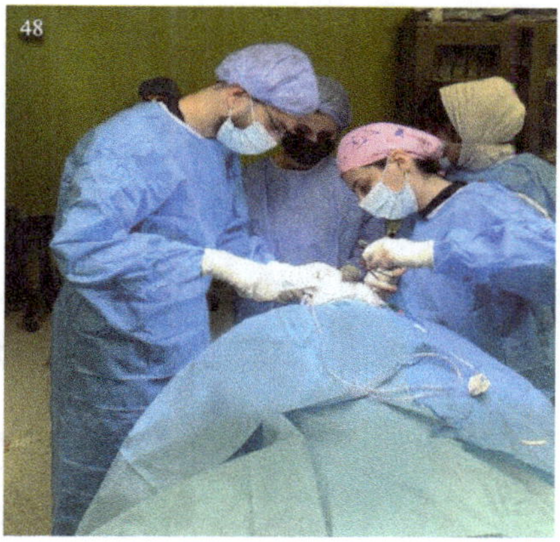

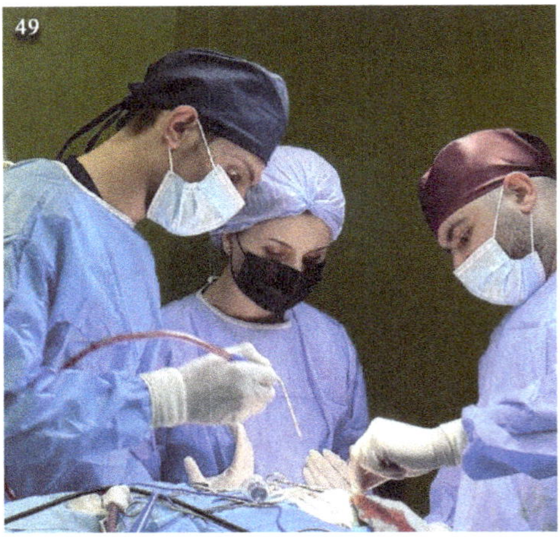
49

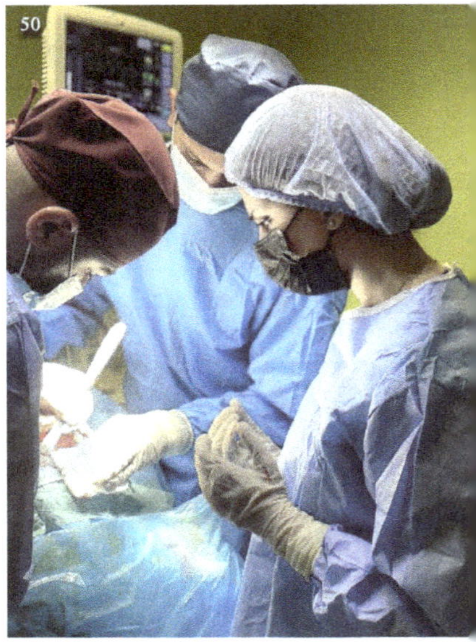
50

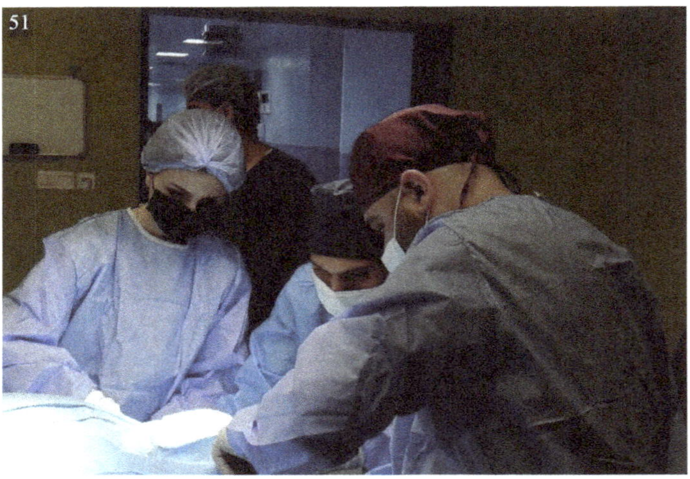
51

Date: February 22, 2022

Occasion: Mentees had the opportunity to observe an endovascular neurosurgical procedure, focusing on catheter-based interventions and neurovascular imaging.

Location: Al-Moayad Private Hospital, Baghdad

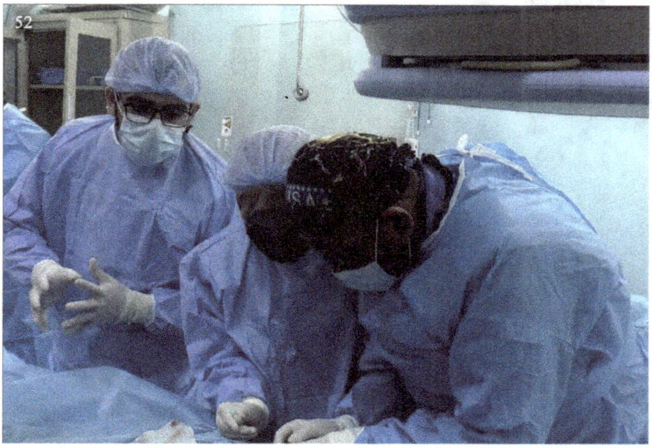

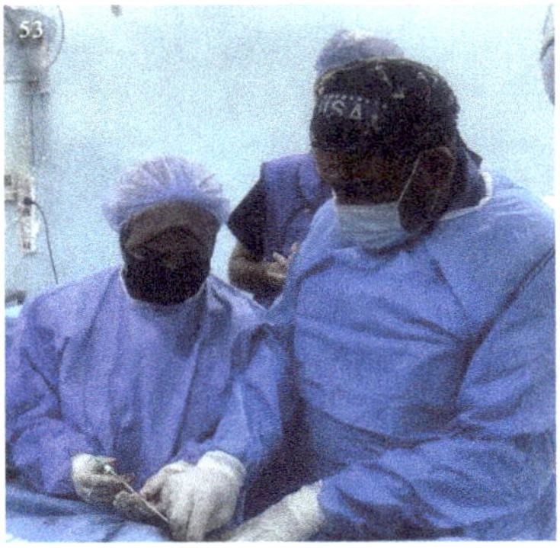

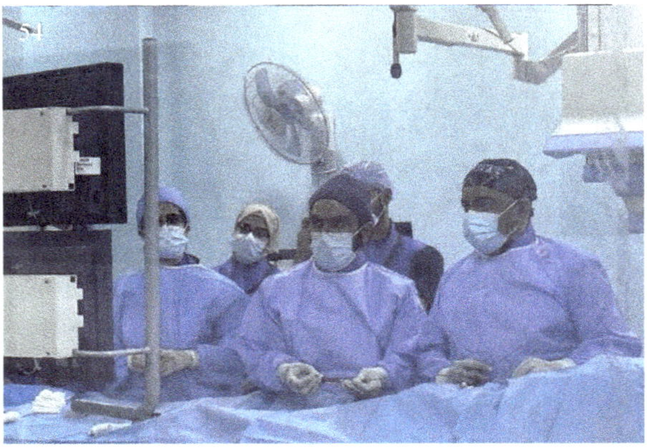

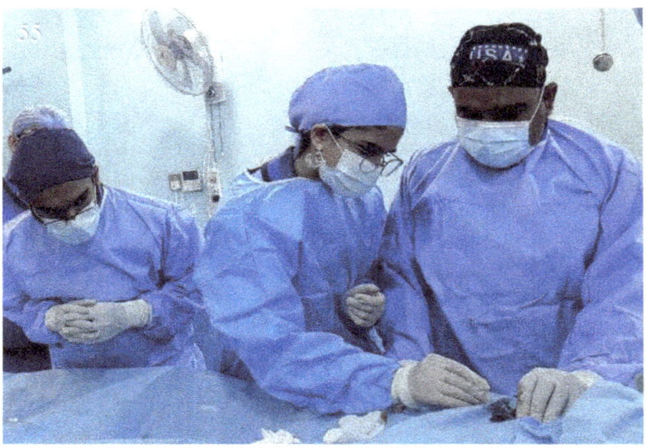

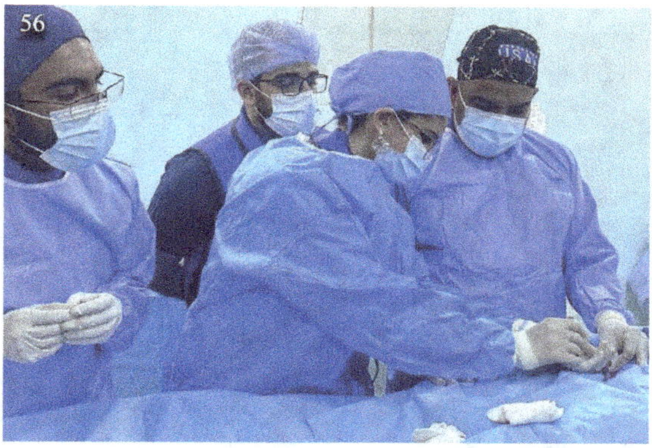

56

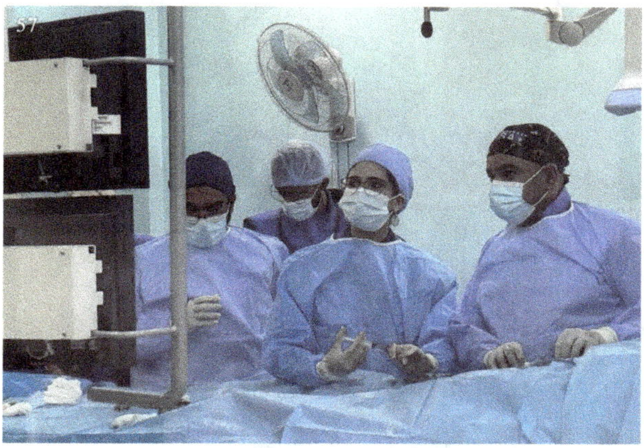

57

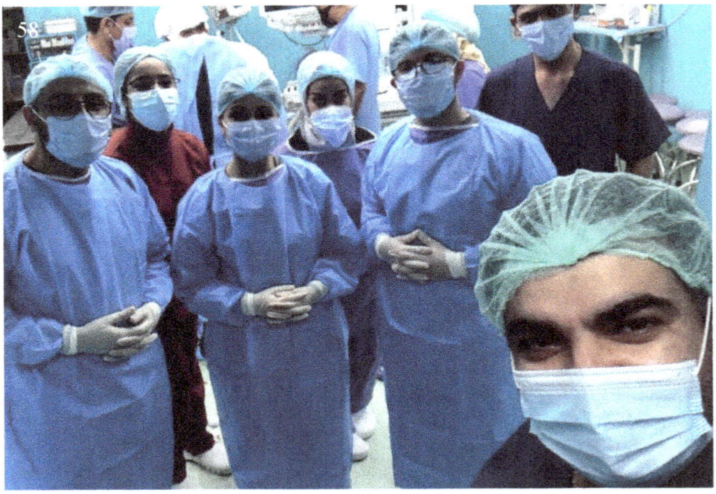
58

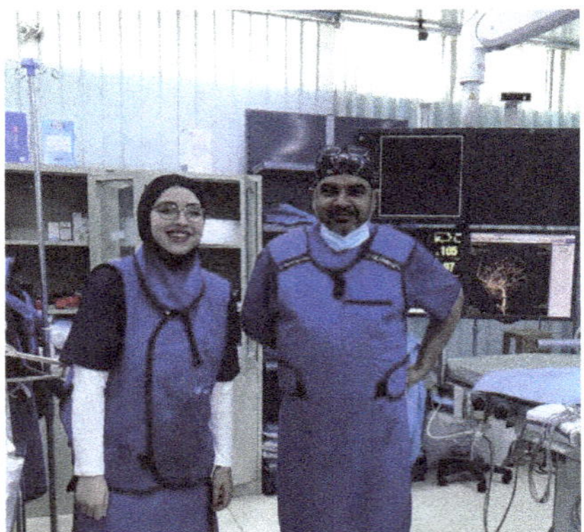

Date: December 1, 2020

Occasion: Mentees had the opportunity to attend a neurosurgical tumor resection procedure, gaining firsthand exposure to intraoperative techniques.

Location: Neurosurgery Teaching Hospital, Baghdad

During this session, mentees observed the excision of a brain tumor, following the step-by-step surgical process. A mentee was given the opportunity to hold the resected tumor, providing a unique educational experience in understanding tumor morphology, texture, and surgical handling. The neurosurgical team explained key principles of tumor removal, hemostasis, and specimen preservation for histopathological analysis.

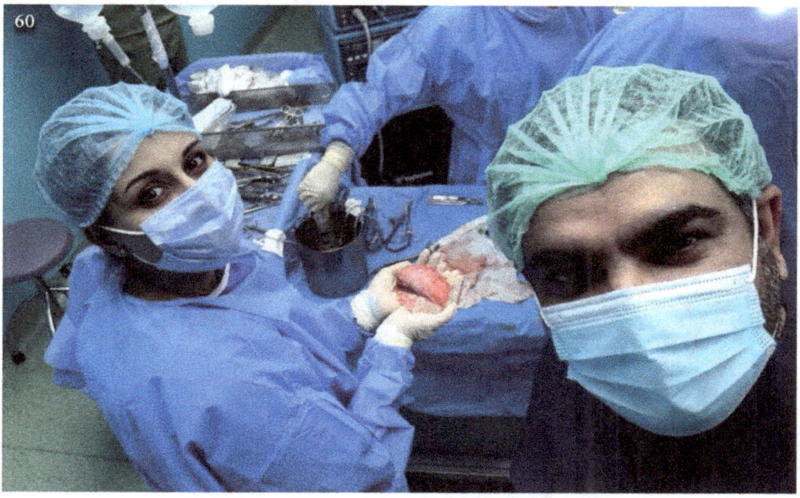

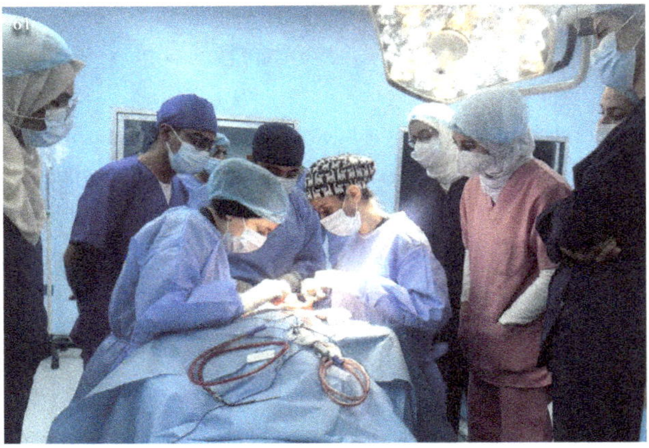

61

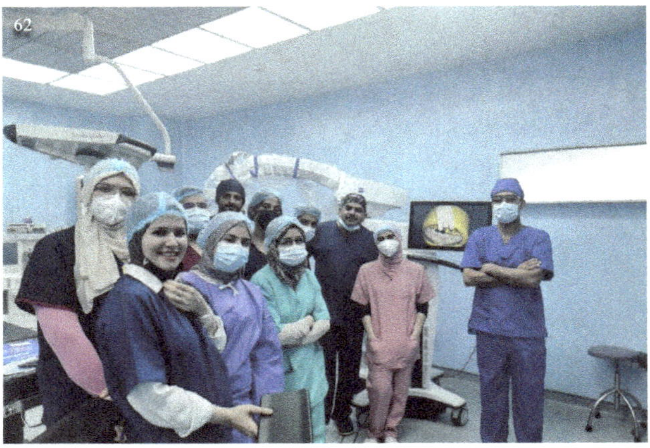

62

Date: June 15, 2021

Occasion: After observing the surgical procedure, mentees engaged in a post-operative debriefing session led by the neurosurgical team. The discussion covered surgical outcomes, intraoperative challenges, and patient prognosis. Mentees had the opportunity to ask questions, analyze imaging findings, and gain insights into decision-making in neurosurgical practice.

Location: Al-Moayad Private Hospital, Baghdad

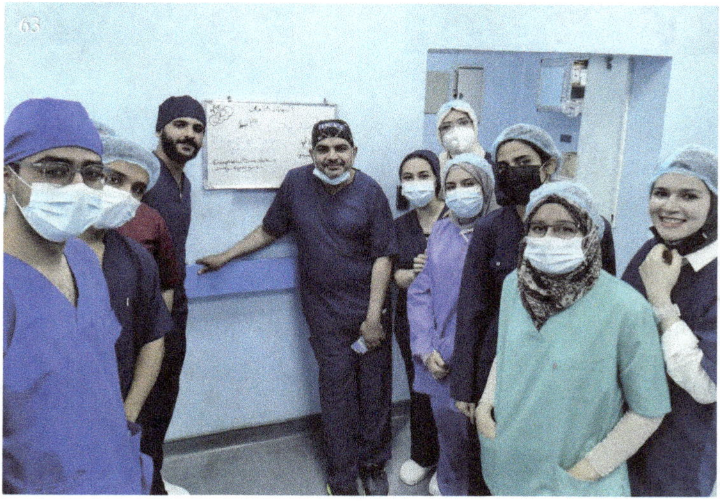

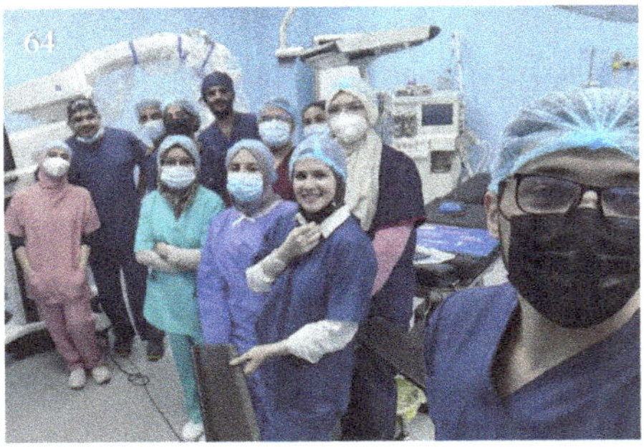
64

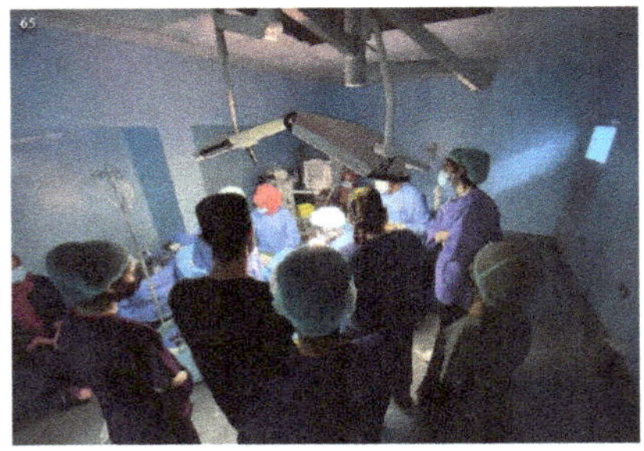
65

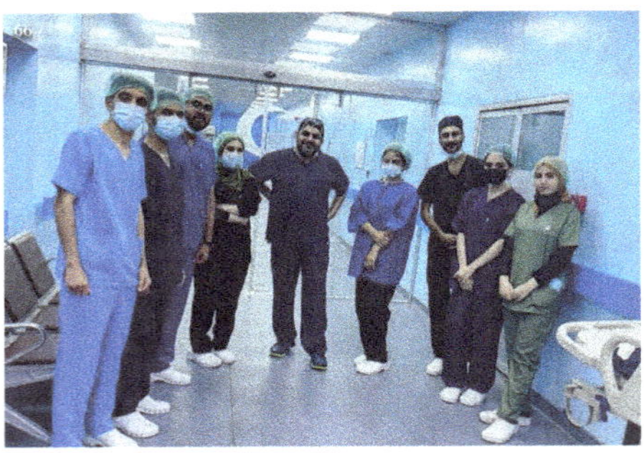
66

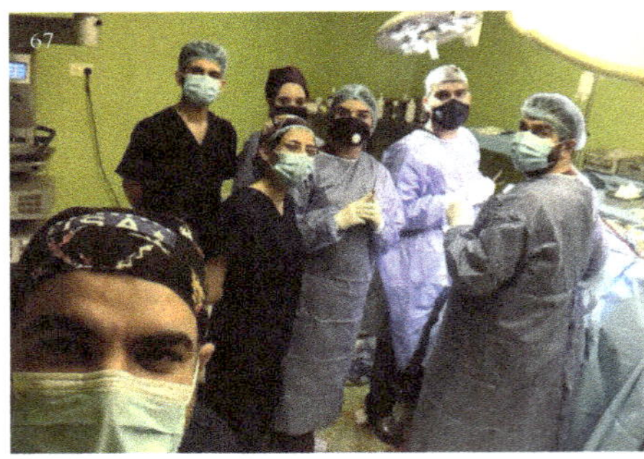
67

Date: July 7, 2021

Occasion: Mentees had the opportunity to observe an **endovascular neurosurgical procedure**, focusing on radiation safety and fluoroscopic imaging techniques.

Location: Al-Moayad Private Hospital, Baghdad

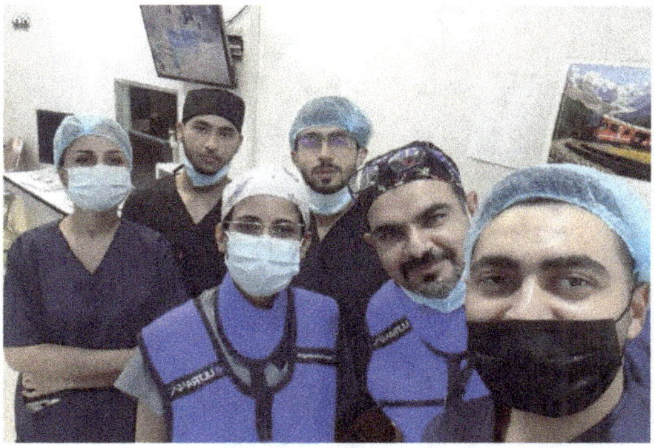

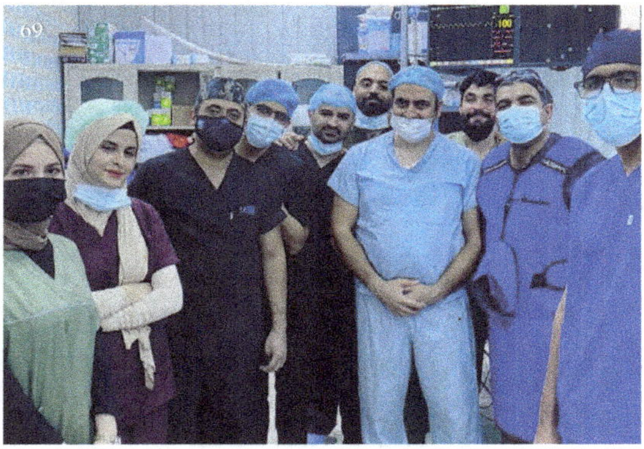

Date: August 20, 2021

Occasion: Mentees had the opportunity to observe a **microsurgical neurosurgical procedure**, gaining insights into high-magnification techniques.

Location: Neurosurgery Teaching Hospital, Baghdad

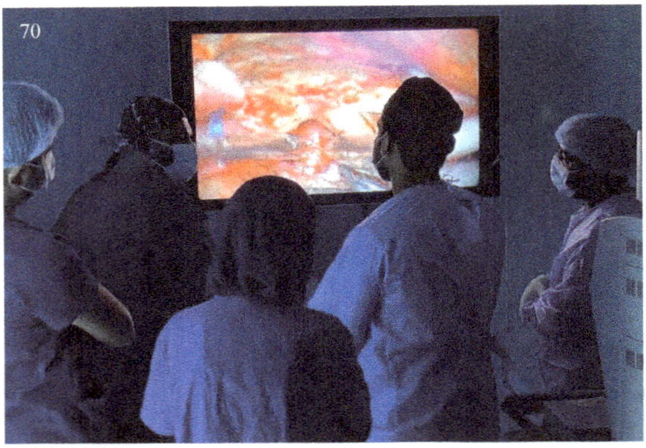

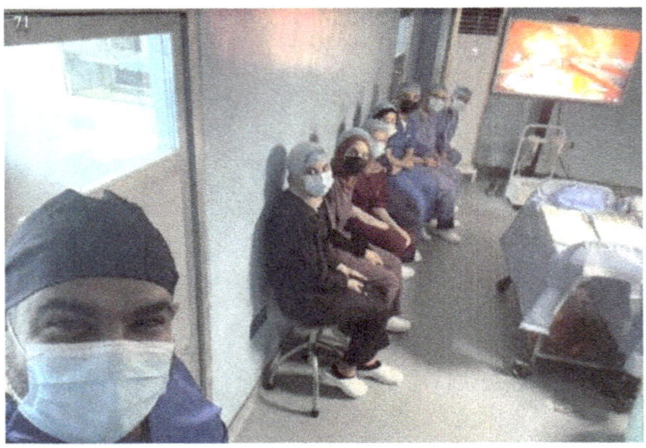

Date: November 8, 2021

Occasion: During this session, mentees observed a minimally invasive endovascular procedure, gaining insights into catheter navigation, real-time angiography, and embolization techniques. The team emphasized radiation safety protocols, including the use of lead aprons, thyroid shields, and appropriate positioning to minimize radiation exposure. The neurosurgeon provided step-by-step explanations, enhancing mentees' understanding of interventional neurovascular techniques.

Location: Al-Moayad Private Hospital, Baghdad

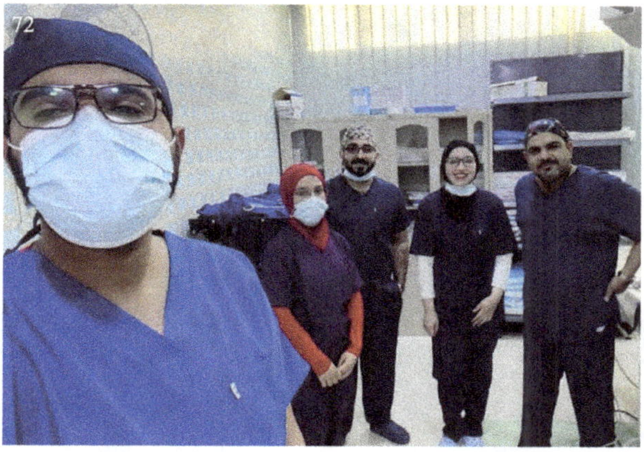

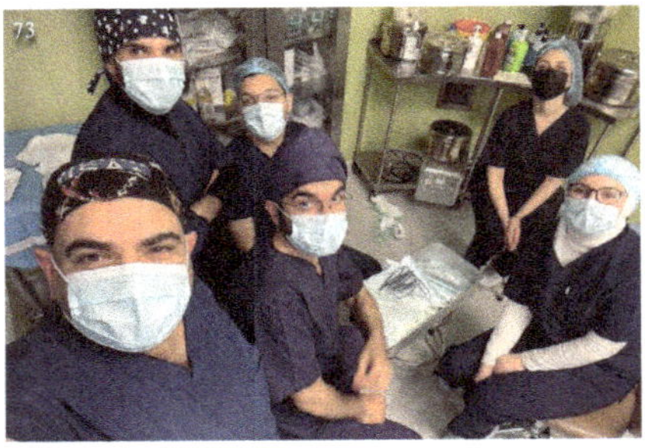
73

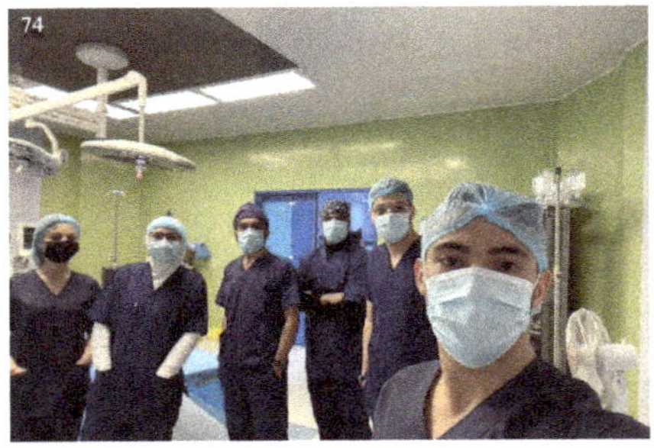
74

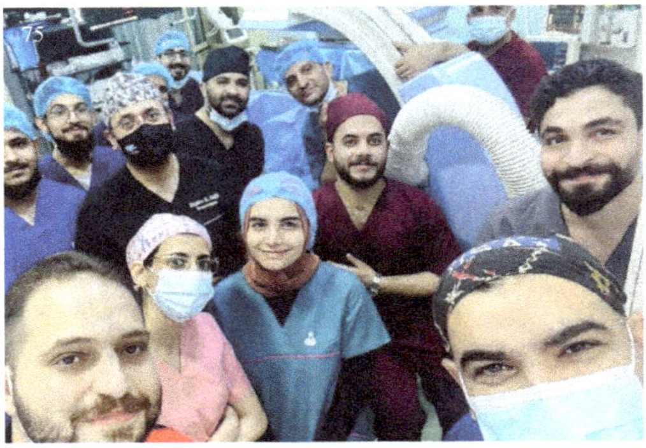
75

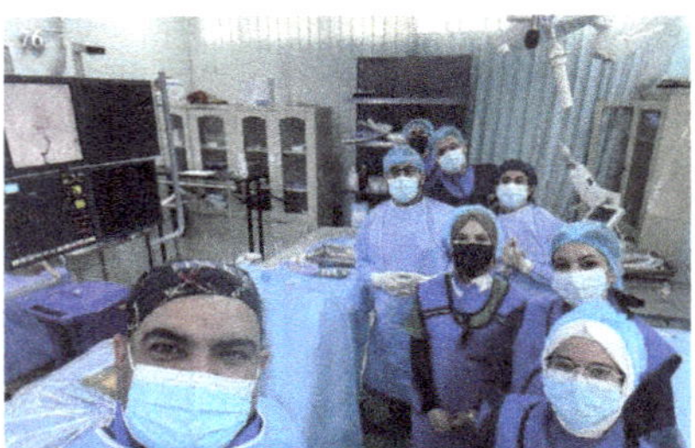
76

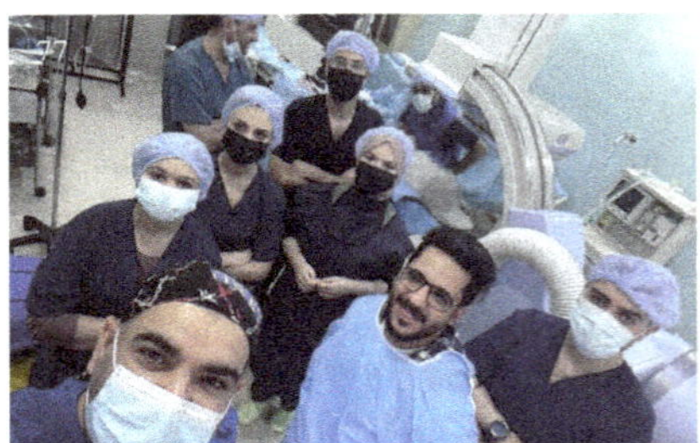

Date: June 15, 2021

Occasion: Mentees had the opportunity to attend the Emergency Department (ED) and Intensive Care Unit (ICU), gaining exposure to acute neurosurgical cases and critical care management.
Location: Neurosurgery Teaching Hospital, Baghdad

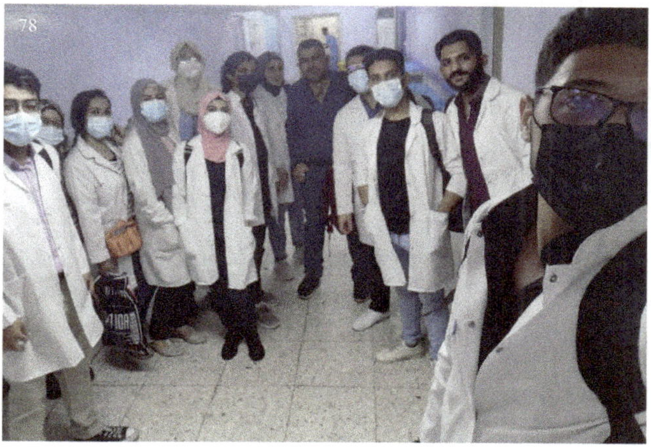

Date: December 4, 2020

Occasion: Mentees had the opportunity to attend a neurosurgical simulation and microsurgical skill lab, focusing on refining their surgical dexterity and understanding of neurosurgical procedures.

Location: Neurosurgery Teaching Hospital, Baghdad

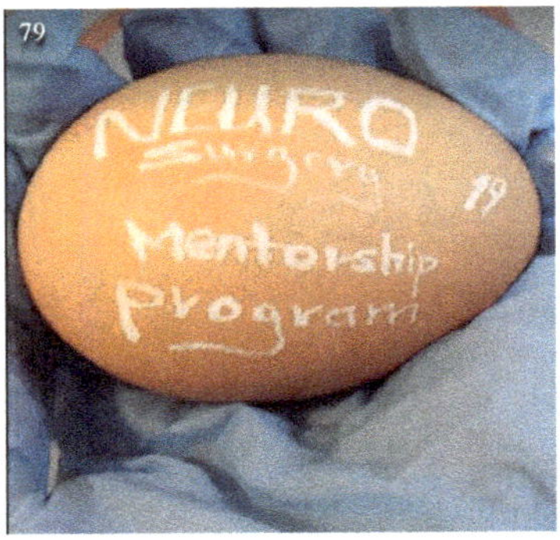

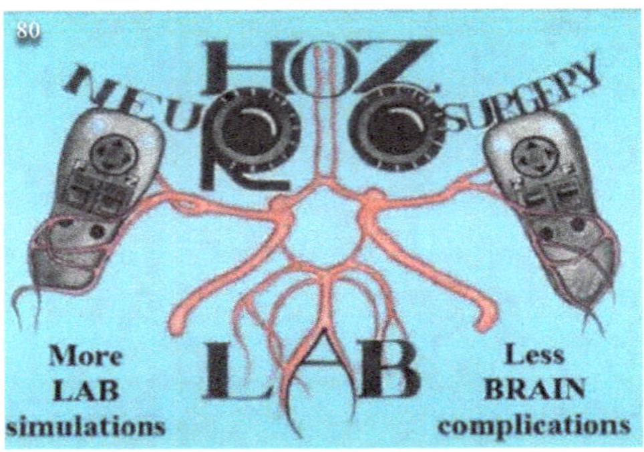

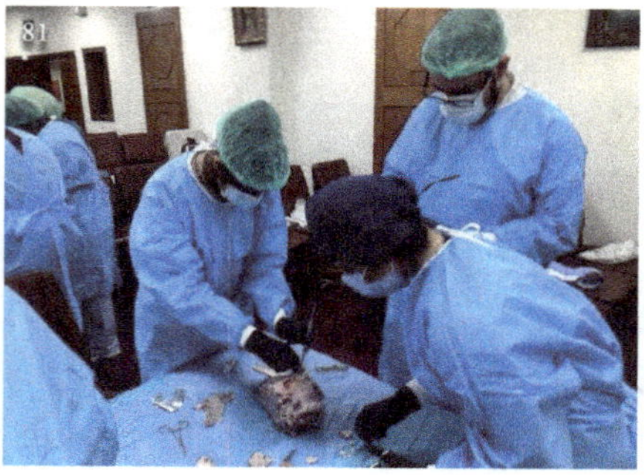

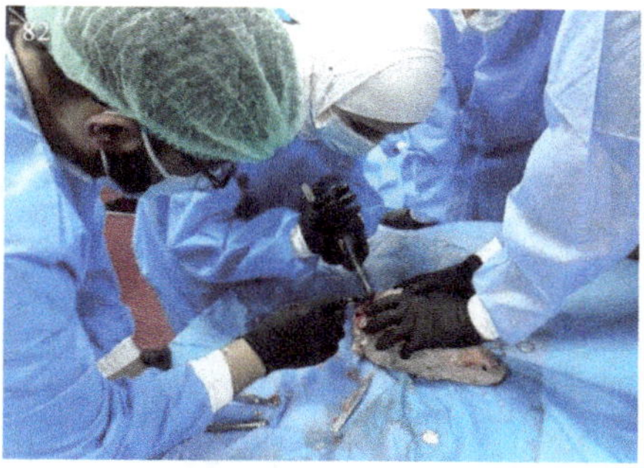

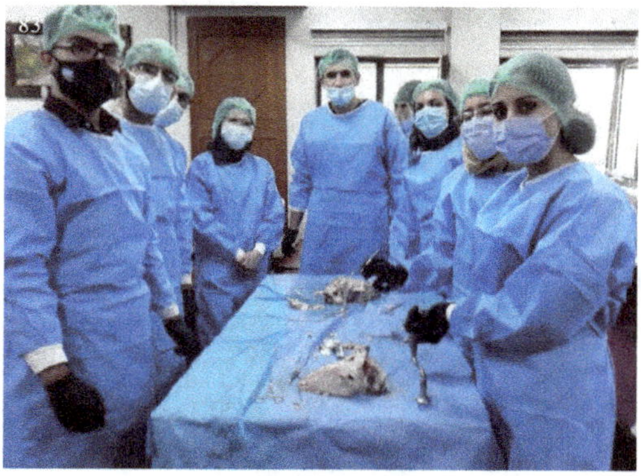

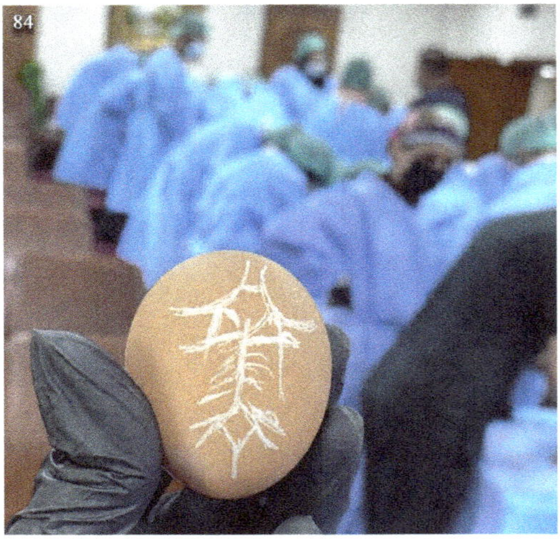

84

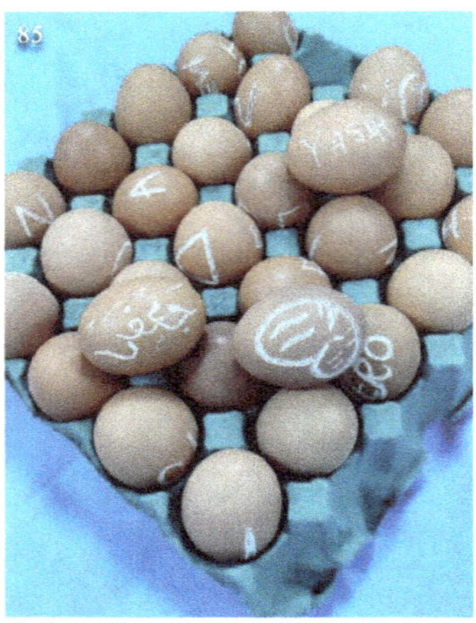

85

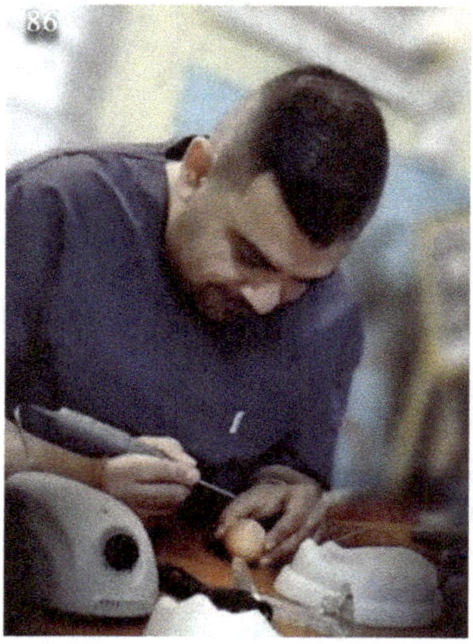

86

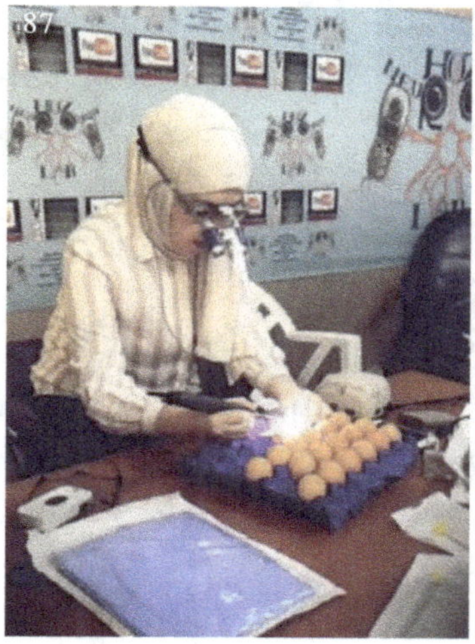

87

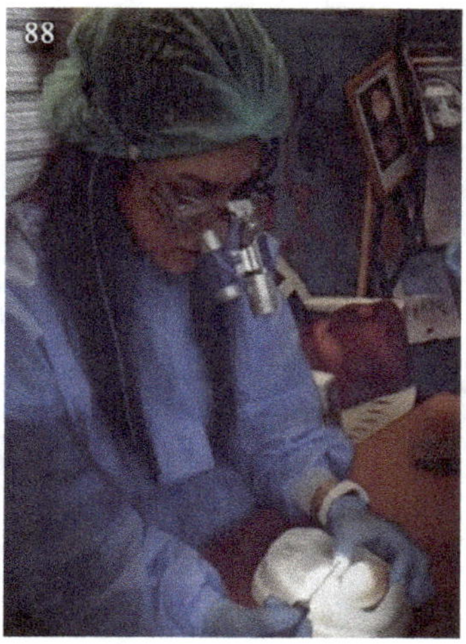

88

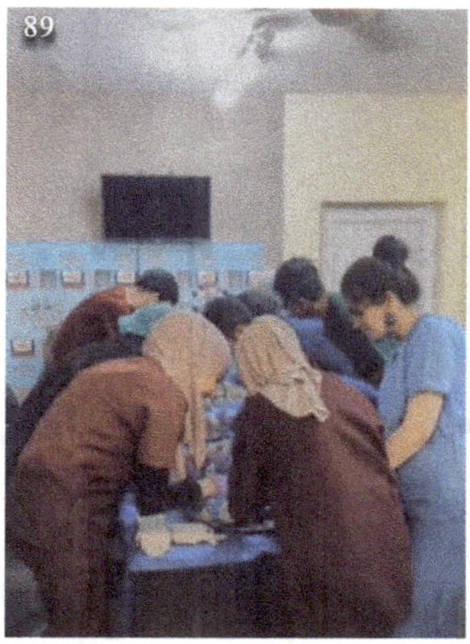

89

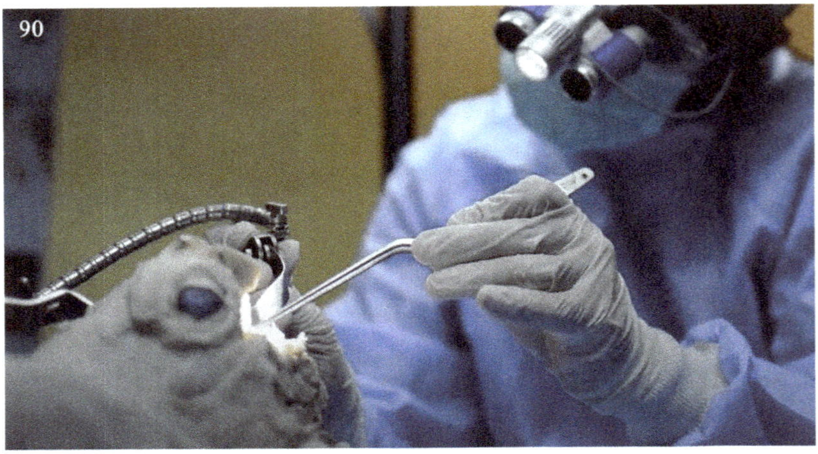

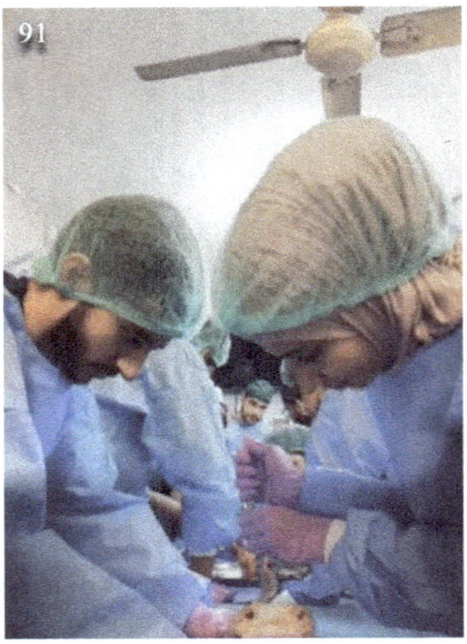

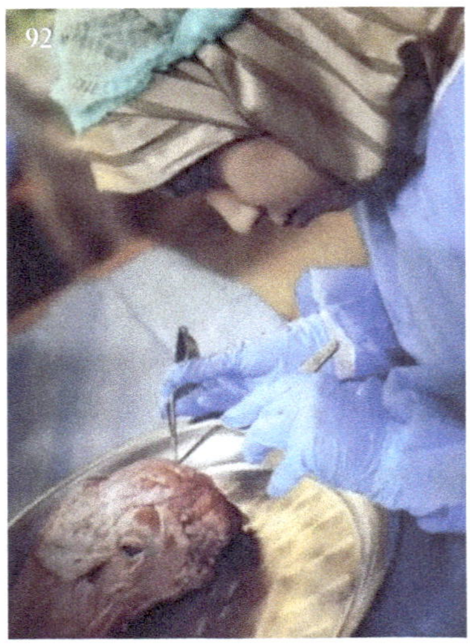

93

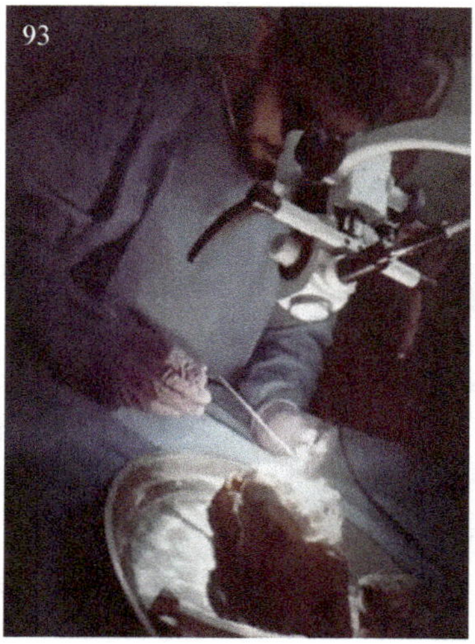

94

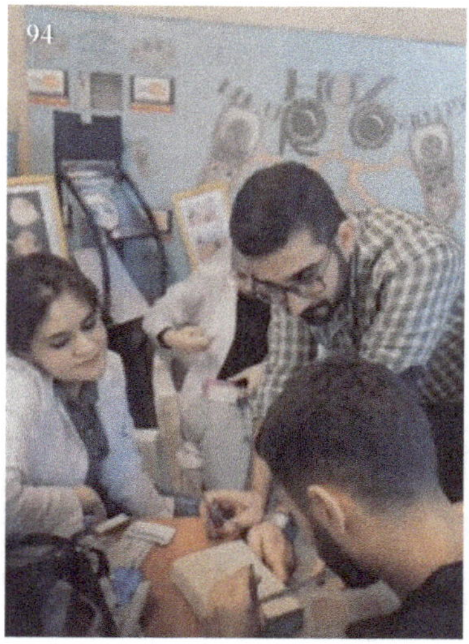

95

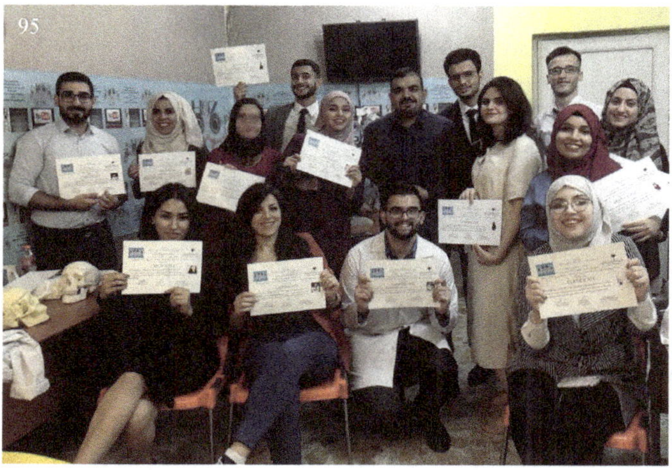

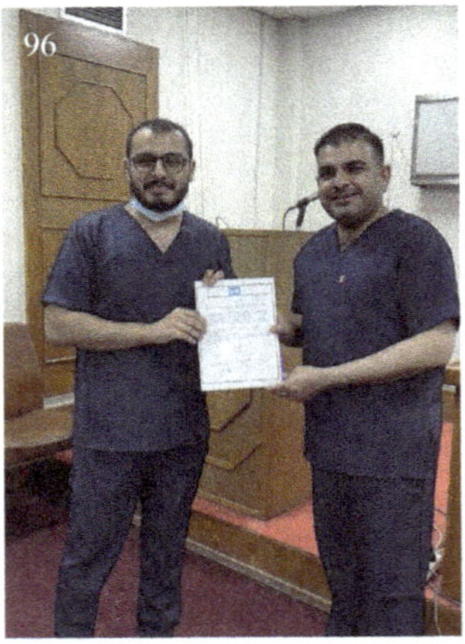
96

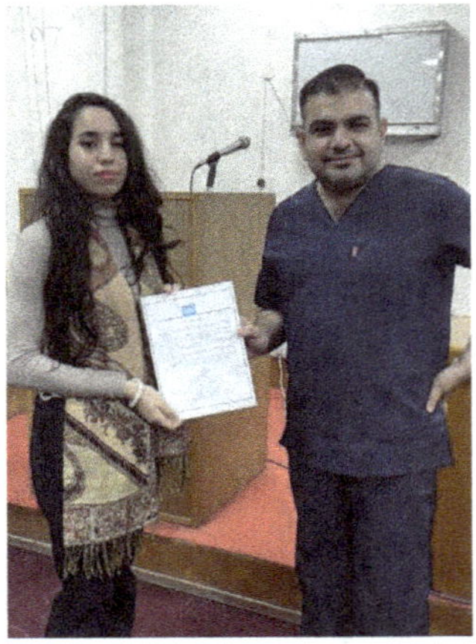

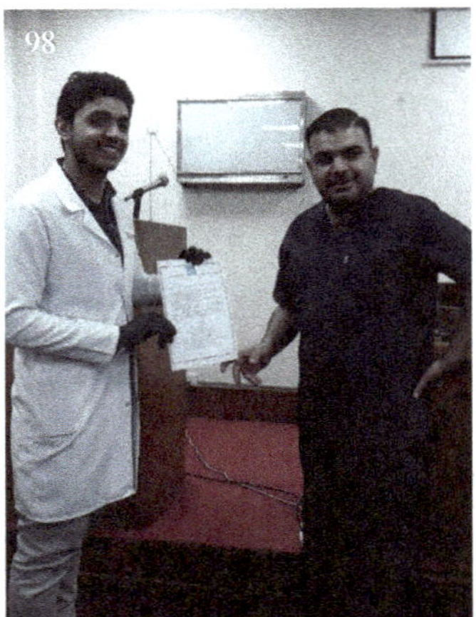
98

Research and Academic Achievements

casion: As part of the mentorship program, mentees had the opportunity to deliver a scientific sentation aimed at improving their academic and communication skills. The session provided nstructive feedback from the mentor, helping them refine their presentation techniques, research clarity, d scientific storytelling.

cation: Online Zoom Meeting

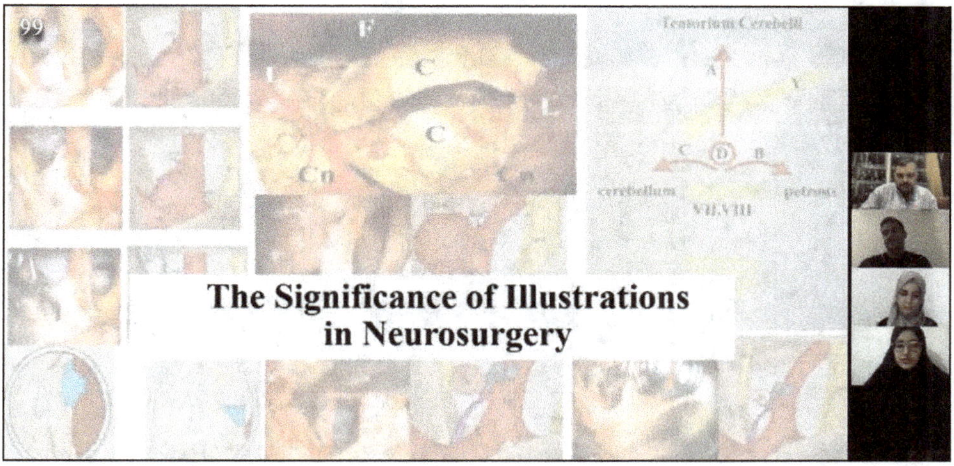

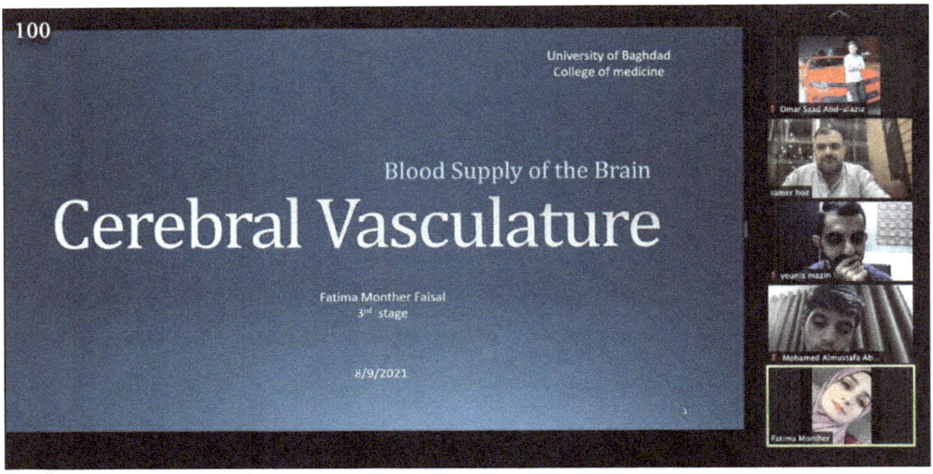
100
University of Baghdad
College of medicine
Blood Supply of the Brain
Cerebral Vasculature
Fatima Monther Faisal
3rd stage
8/9/2021

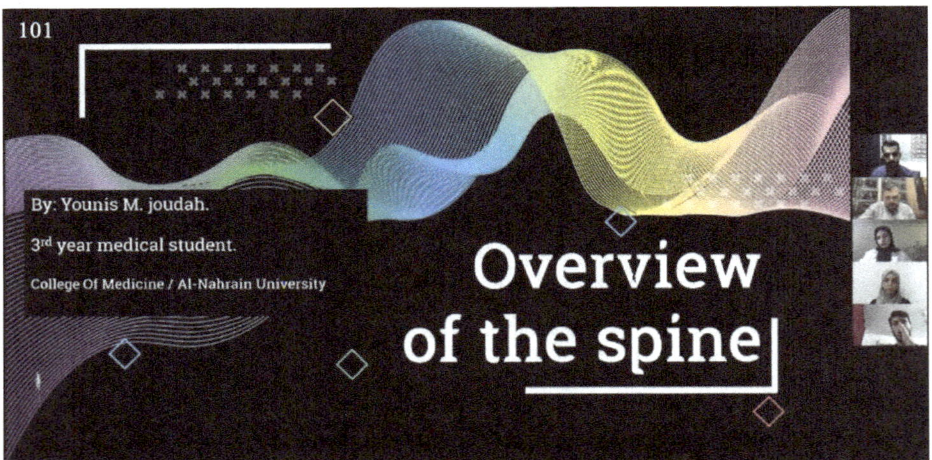
101
By: Younis M. joudah.
3rd year medical student.
College Of Medicine / Al-Nahrain University
Overview
of the spine

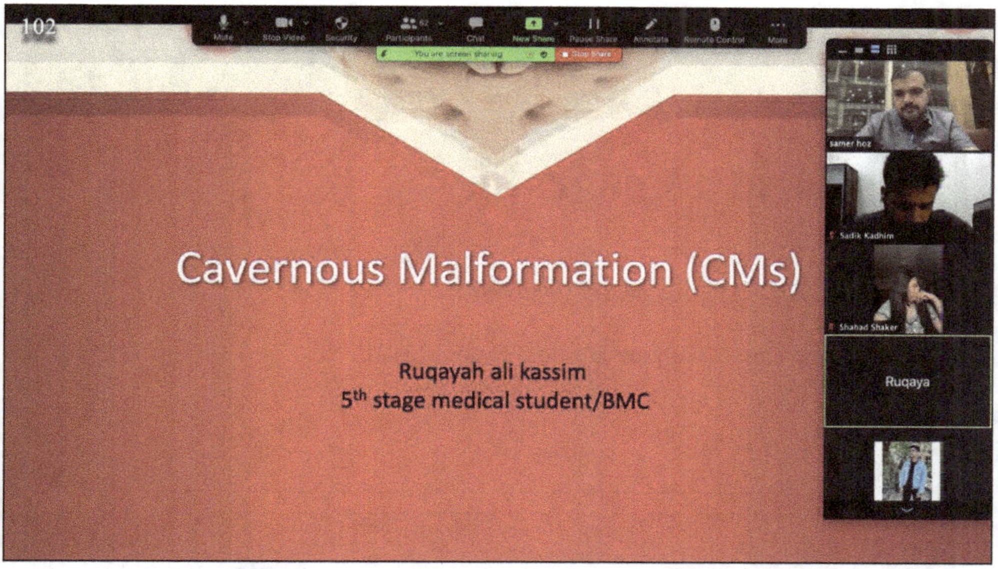
102
Cavernous Malformation (CMs)
Ruqayah ali kassim
5th stage medical student/BMC
samer hoz
Sadik Kadhim
Shahad Shaker
Ruqaya

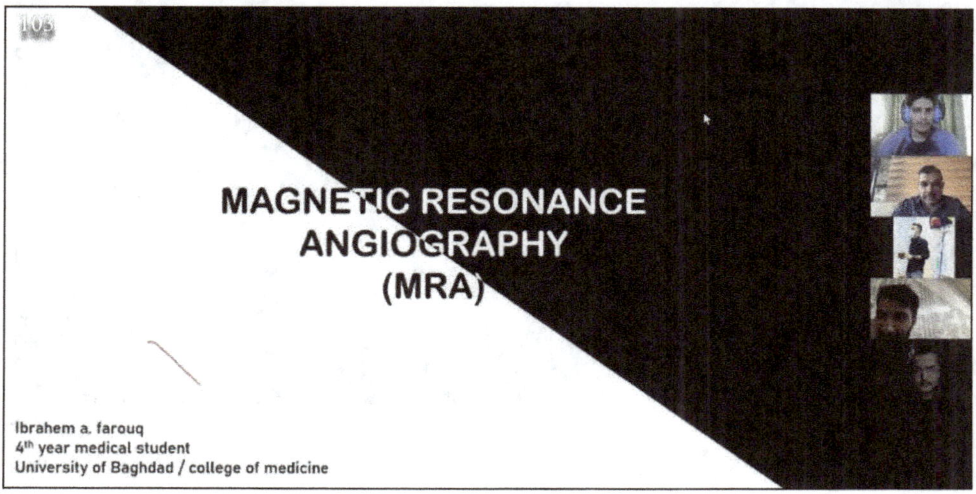
103
MAGNETIC RESONANCE
ANGIOGRAPHY
(MRA)
Ibrahem a. farouq
4th year medical student
University of Baghdad / college of medicine

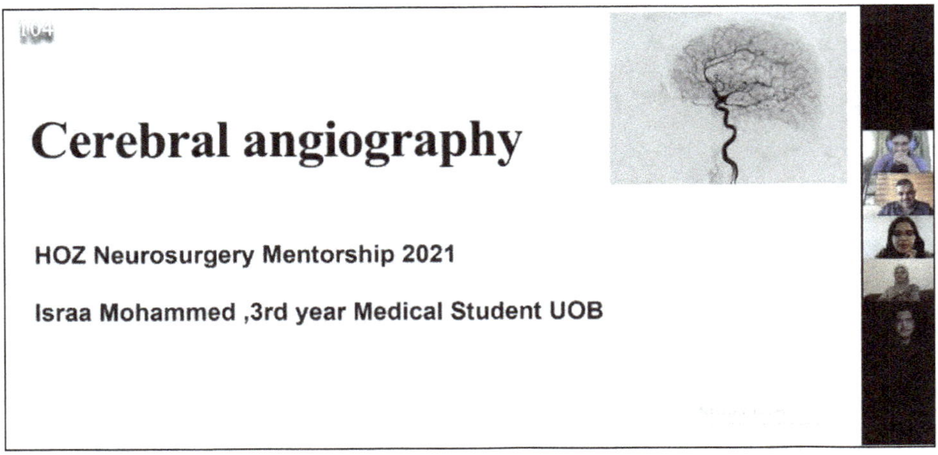
104
Cerebral angiography
HOZ Neurosurgery Mentorship 2021
Israa Mohammed ,3rd year Medical Student UOB

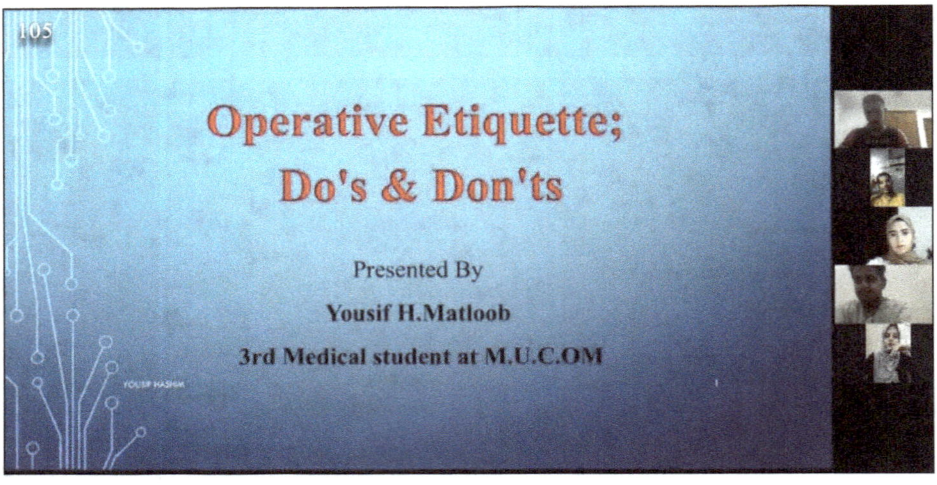
105
Operative Etiquette;
Do's & Don'ts
Presented By
Yousif H.Matloob
3rd Medical student at M.U.C.OM

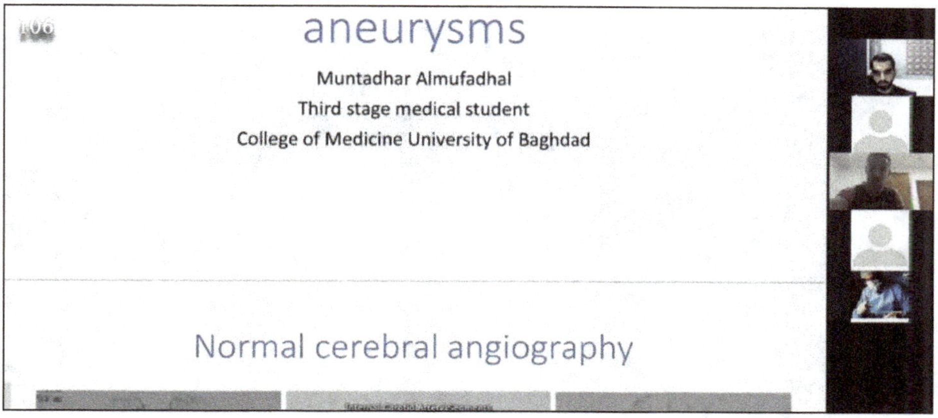
106
aneurysms
Muntadhar Almufadhal
Third stage medical student
College of Medicine University of Baghdad
Normal cerebral angiography

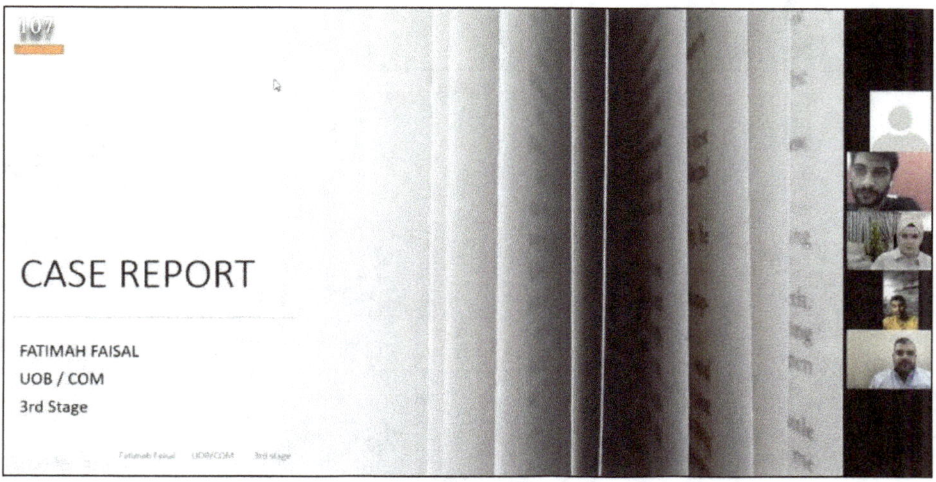
107
CASE REPORT
FATIMAH FAISAL
UOB / COM
3rd Stage

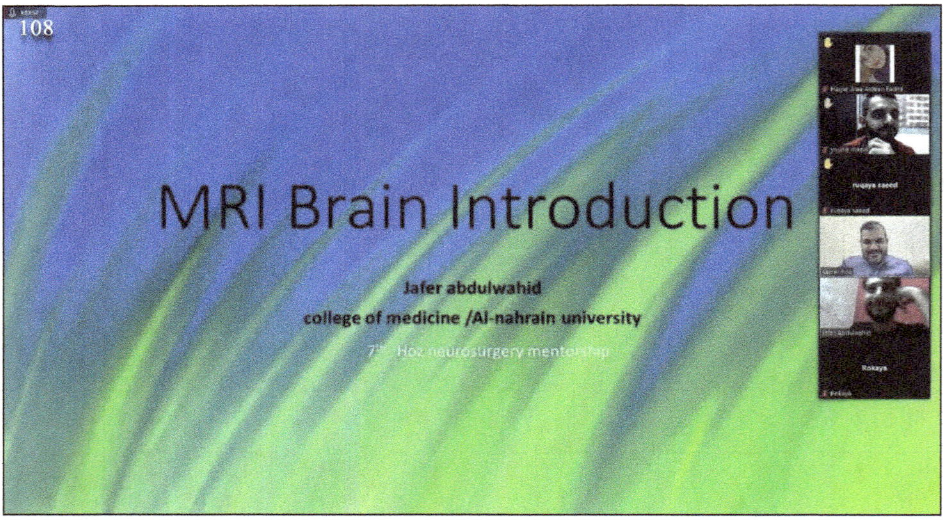
108
MRI Brain Introduction
Jafer abdulwahid
college of medicine /Al-nahrain university
7th Hoz neurosurgery mentorship

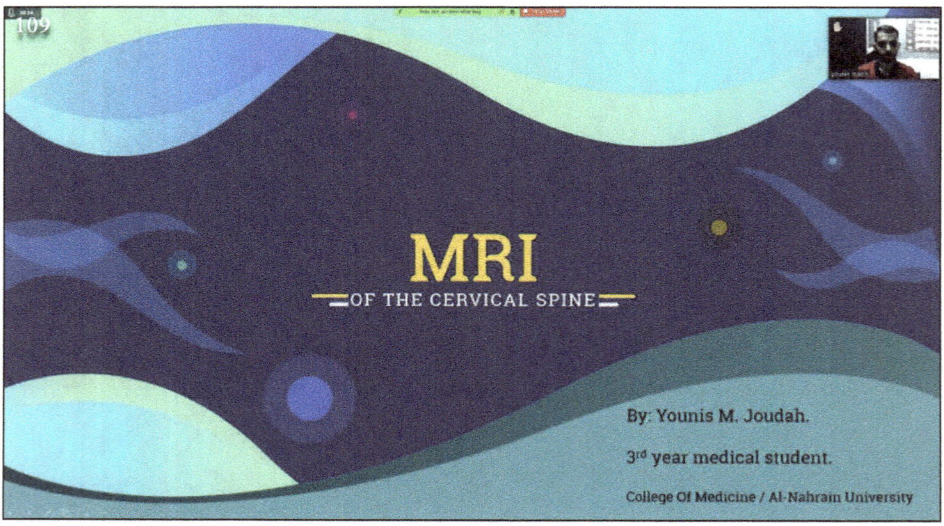
109
MRI
OF THE CERVICAL SPINE
By: Younis M. Joudah.
3rd year medical student.
College Of Medicine / Al-Nahrain University

110

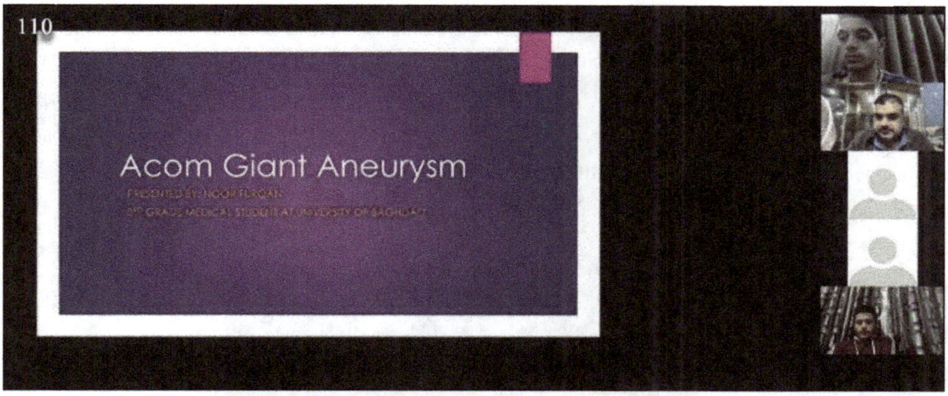
Acom Giant Aneurysm

111

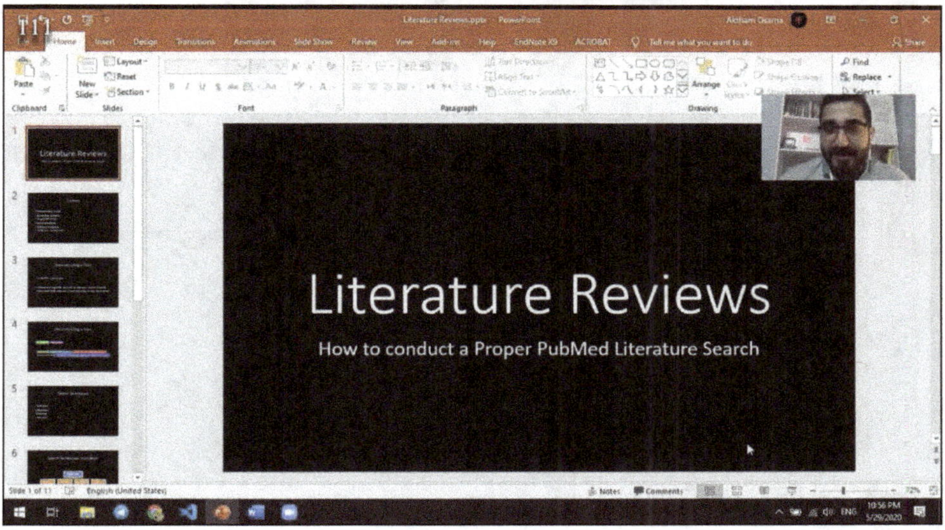
Literature Reviews
How to conduct a Proper PubMed Literature Search

Date: December 9, 2021

Occasion: A collaborative initiative between the Baghdad Neurosurgery Team and the California School of Medicine, in partnership with Surgical Neurology International (SNI). The session was the first round of discussions focusing on the fundamentals of designing and developing a research project in clinical neurosciences.Participants engaged in discussions led by **Dr. Jorge A. Lazareff**, a distinguished professor of neurosurgery from the University of California, Los Angeles

Location: Online Zoom Meeting

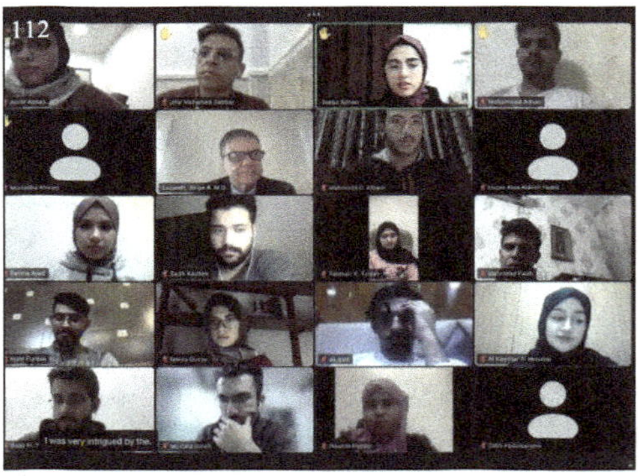

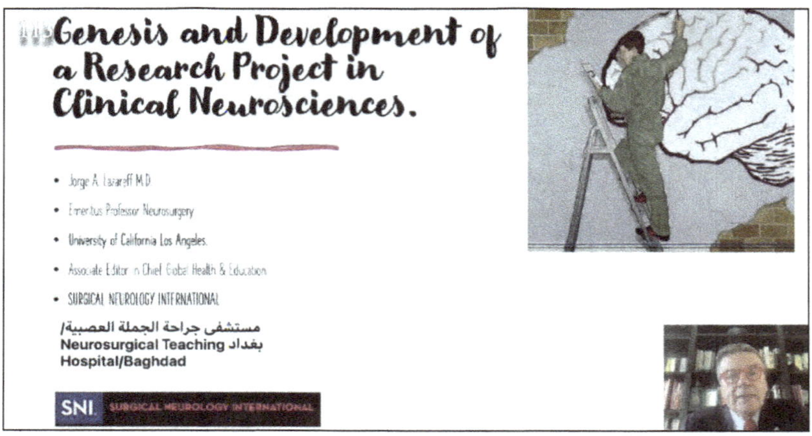

International Collaborations and Special Guests

Date: December 9, 2020

Occasion: As part of the mentorship program, medical students had the opportunity to present their work on Neurosurgical TV Live, engaging with an international audience of experts and researchers. This session was an important step in enhancing mentees' confidence and visibility in the field of neurosurgery, and fostering future collaborations and research endeavors.

Location: Online Zoom Meeting – Neurosurgical TV Live

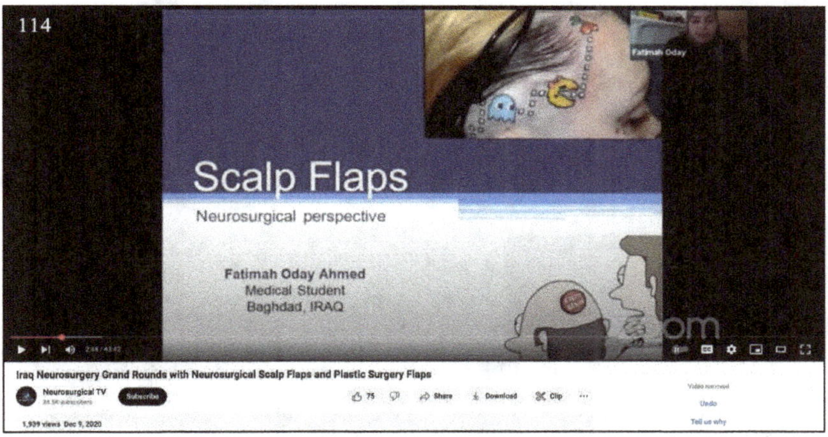

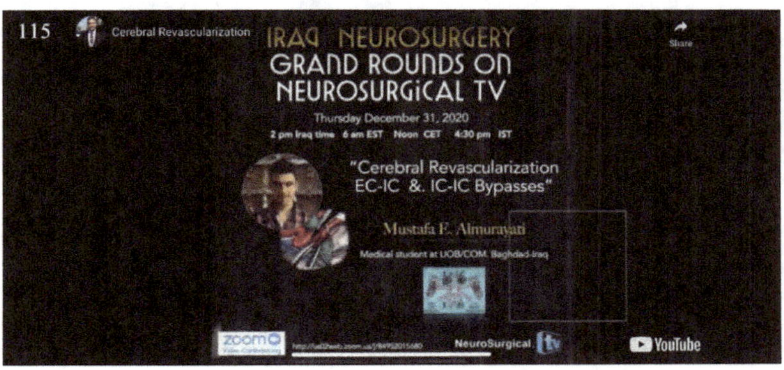

Date: June 7th, 2021

Occasion: As part of the mentorship program, a collaborative Zoom meeting was held with special guests, including Dr. Faisal, who shared insights on his personal experience and journey in international medical residency. This event provided mentees with first-hand knowledge on navigating the residency application process and career development strategies in an international setting.

Location: Online Zoom Meeting

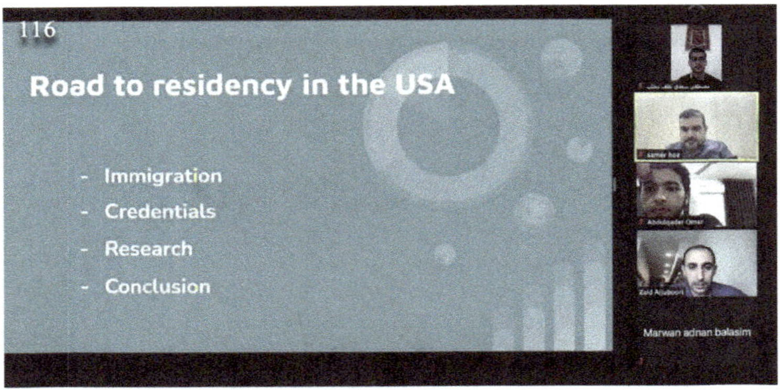

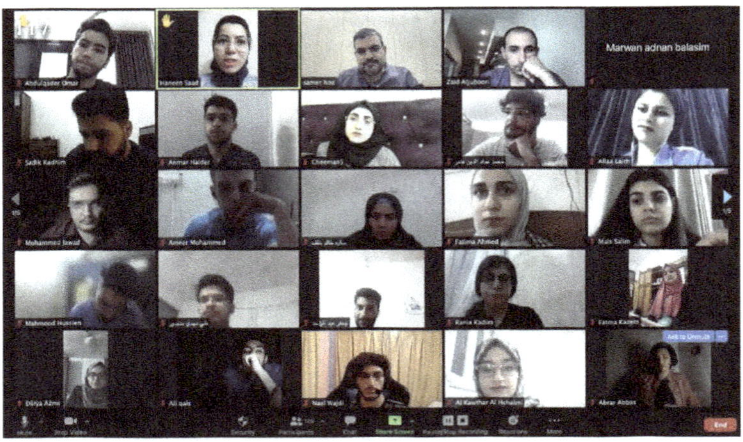

Date: June 7th, 2021

Occasion: As part of the mentorship program, a **collaborative Zoom meeting** was held with special guest **Dr. Osama Al-Awadi**, who shared his **personal journey and experiences** in the field.

Location: Online Zoom Meeting

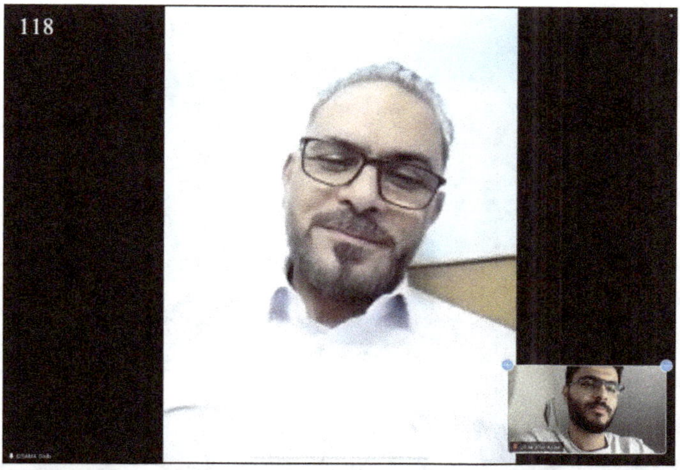

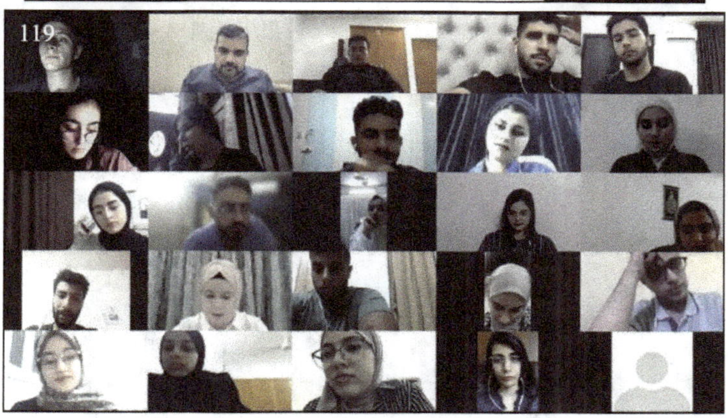

Date: June 7th, 2021

Occasion: As part of the mentorship program, a collaborative Zoom meeting was conducted with special guest Dr. Margarida Gocieça, who shared her expert insights and experiences with aspiring neurosurgeons.

Location: Online Zoom Meeting

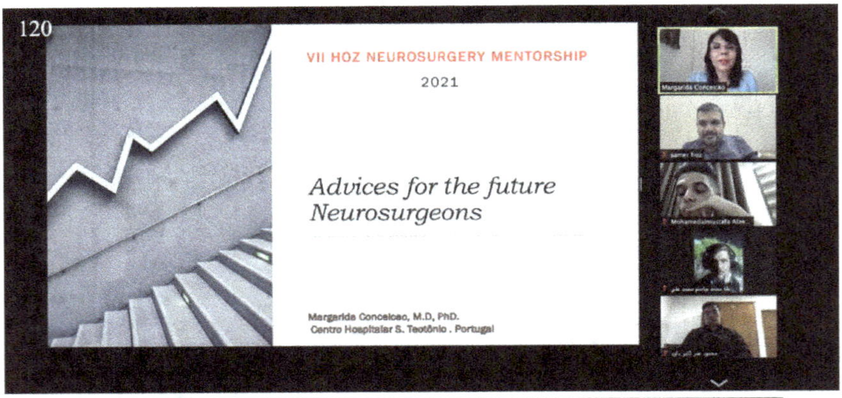

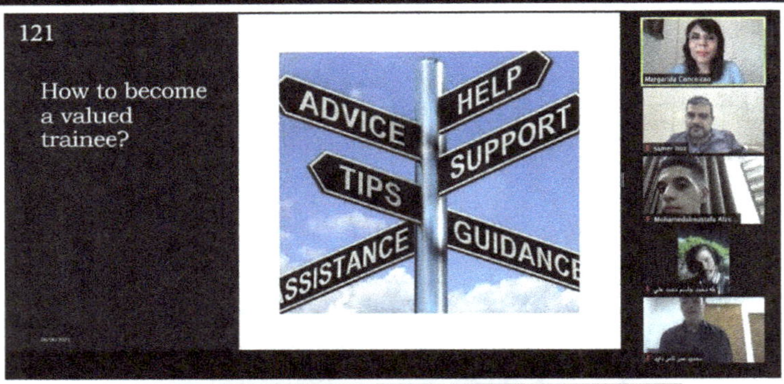

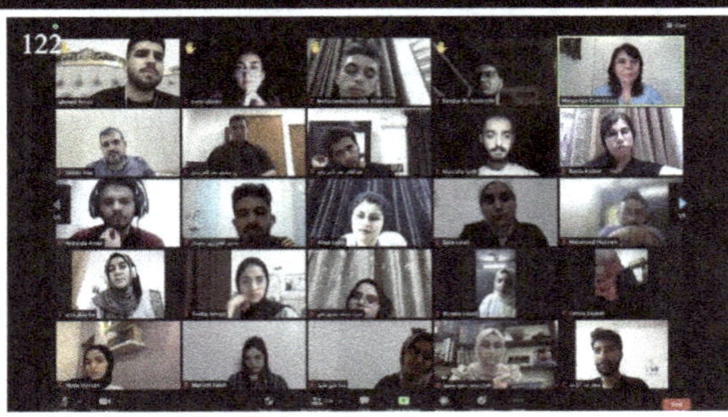

Date: September 27th, 2021

Occasion: As part of the mentorship program, a collaborative Zoom meeting was conducted with special guest **Dr. Elena Neştian**, who shared her expert insights and experiences with aspiring neurosurgeons.

Location: Online Zoom Meeting

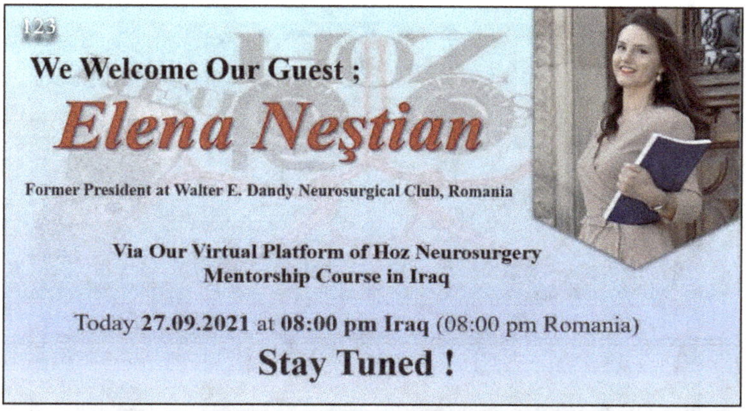
123
We Welcome Our Guest ;
Elena Neştian
Former President at Walter E. Dandy Neurosurgical Club, Romania
Via Our Virtual Platform of Hoz Neurosurgery
Mentorship Course in Iraq
Today 27.09.2021 at 08:00 pm Iraq (08:00 pm Romania)
Stay Tuned !

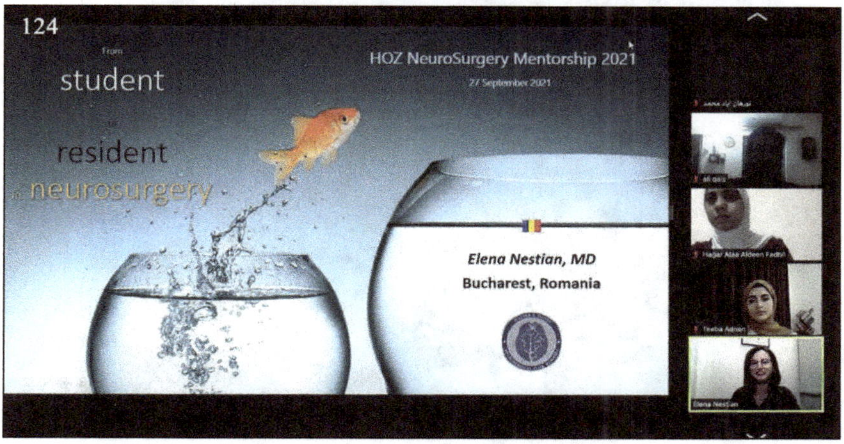

Date: September 27th, 2021

Occasion: As part of the mentorship program, a collaborative Zoom meeting was conducted with special gue **Dr. Esene**, who shared his expert insights and experiences with aspiring neurosurgeon

Location: Online Zoom Meeting

125

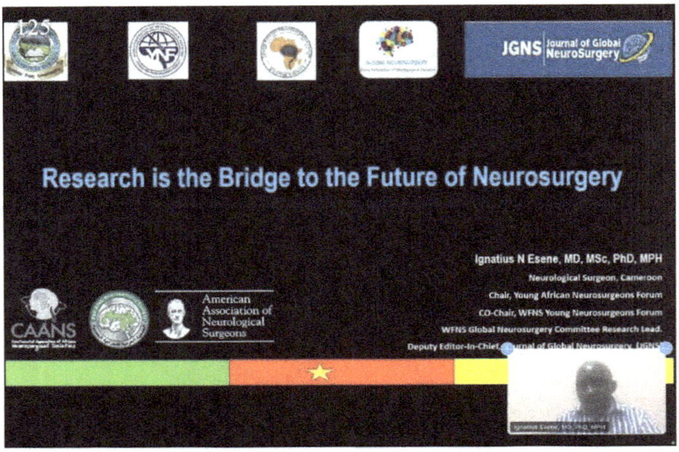

126

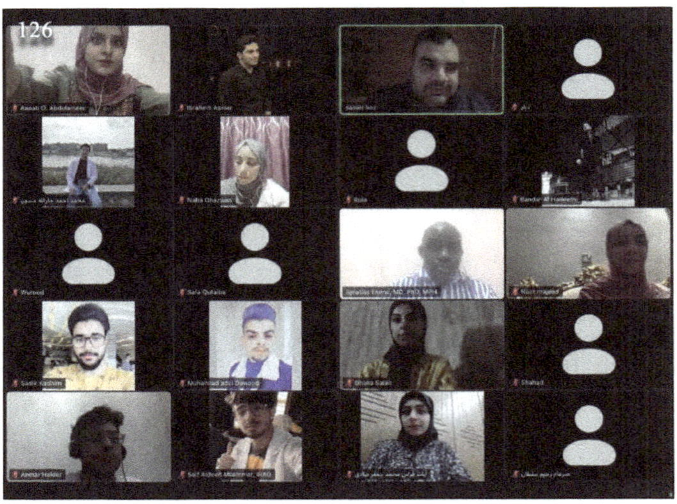

Date: October 3rd, 2021

Occasion: As part of the mentorship program, a collaborative Zoom meeting was conducted with special guest **Dr. Ghayath**, who shared his expert insights and experiences with aspiring neurosurgeons.

Location: Online Zoom Meeting

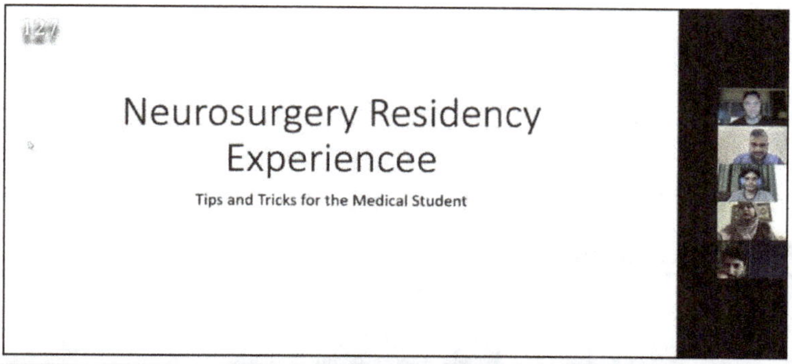

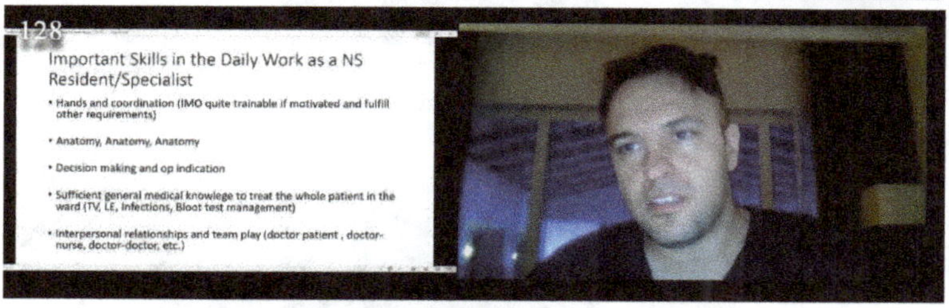

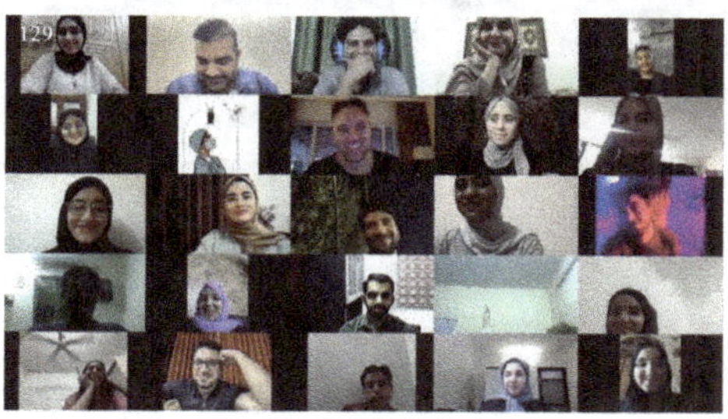

Date: January 16th, 2022

Occasion: As part of the mentorship program, a collaborative Zoom meeting was conducted with Surgical Neurology International (SNI), focusing on guidance, mentorship, and advancements in neurosurgery.

Location: Online Zoom Meeting

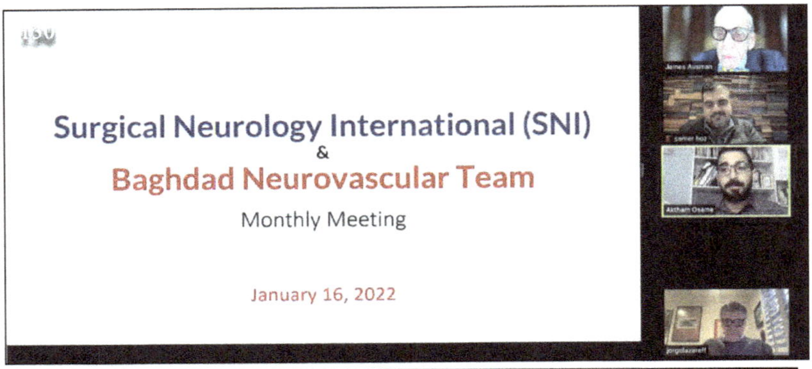
Surgical Neurology International (SNI)
&
Baghdad Neurovascular Team
Monthly Meeting
January 16, 2022

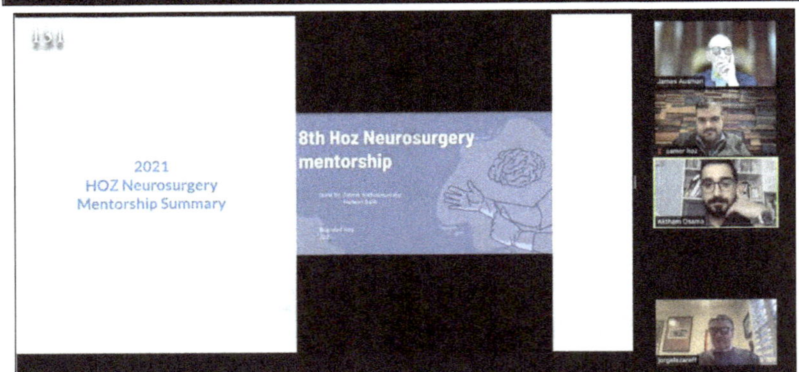

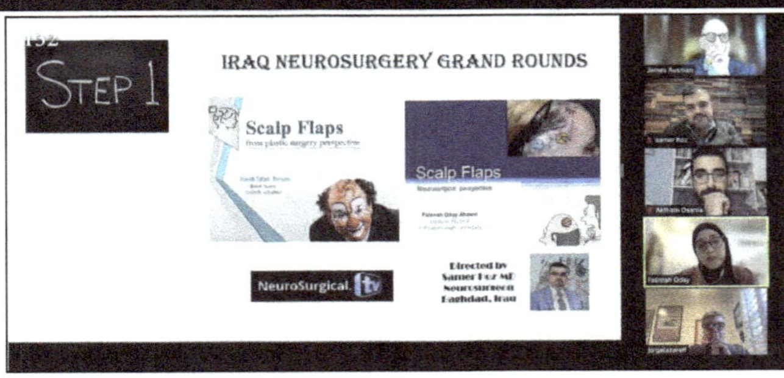

Date: September 8th, 2021

Occasion: The first online mentorship meeting with Dr. Hosam, where the mentor facilitated a collaborative Zoom session to discuss key aspects of neurosurgical mentorship and professional development.

Location: Online Zoom Meeting

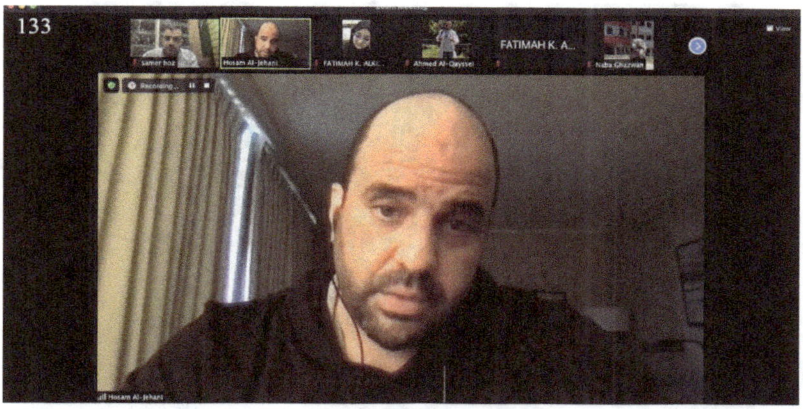

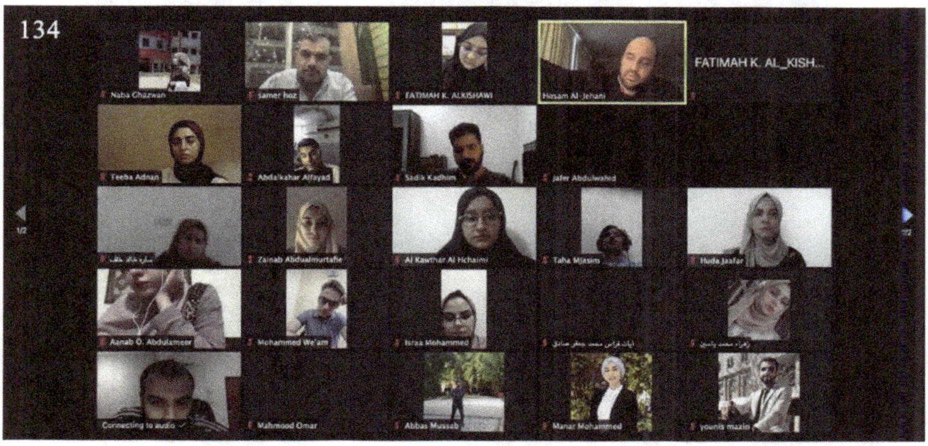

Date: April 23rd, 2021

Occasion: Collaboration with UpSurgeon

Location: Online Zoom Meeting and Neurosurgery Teaching Hospital.

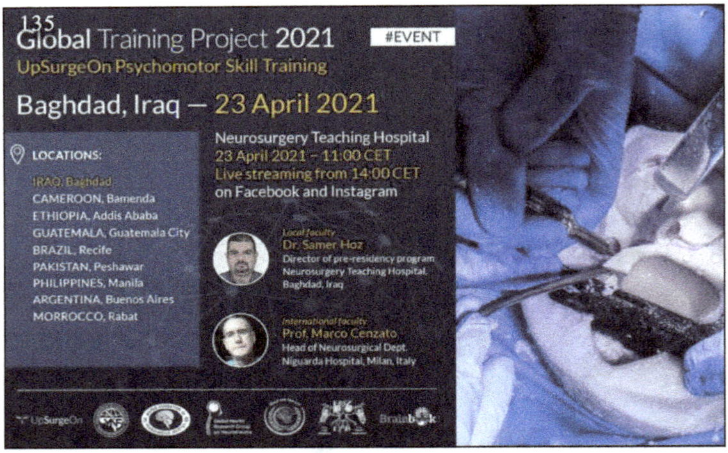

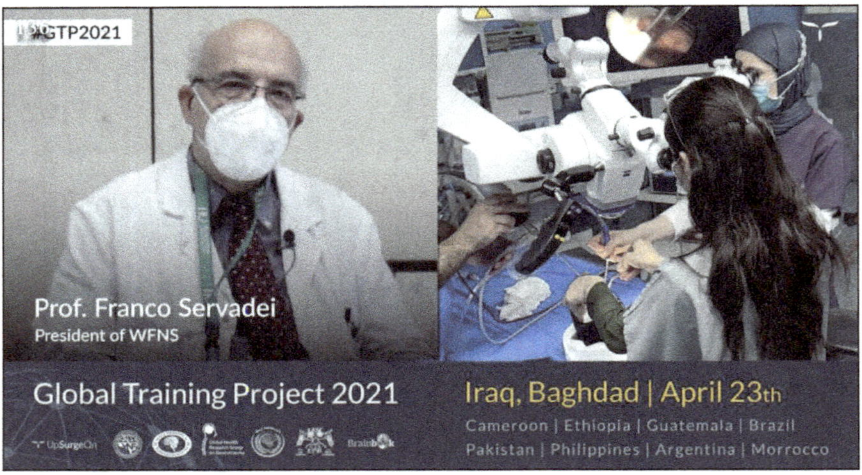

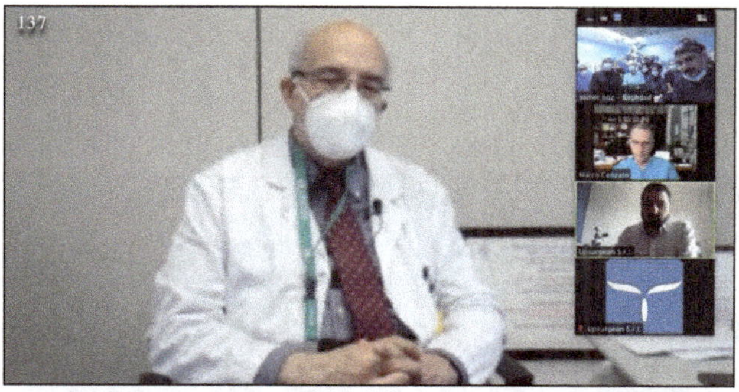
137

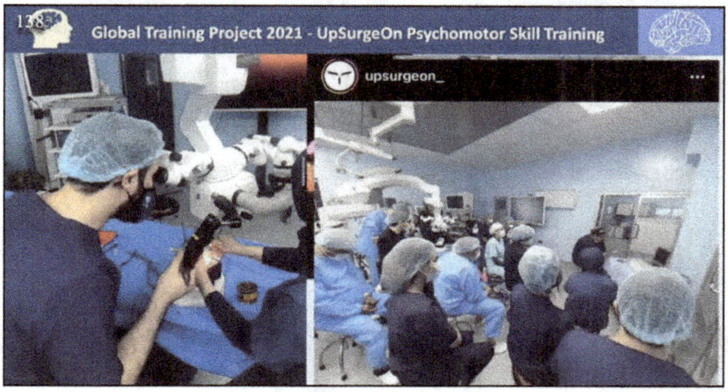
138
Global Training Project 2021 - UpSurgeOn Psychomotor Skill Training
upsurgeon_

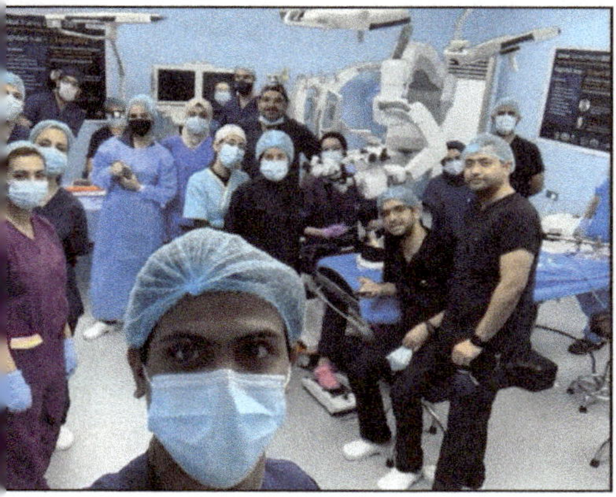

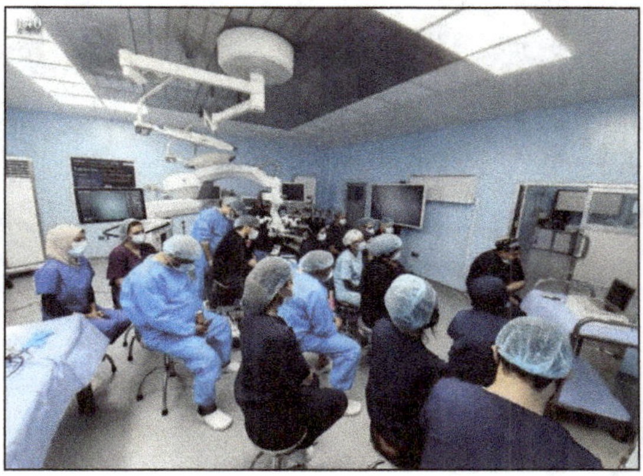
140

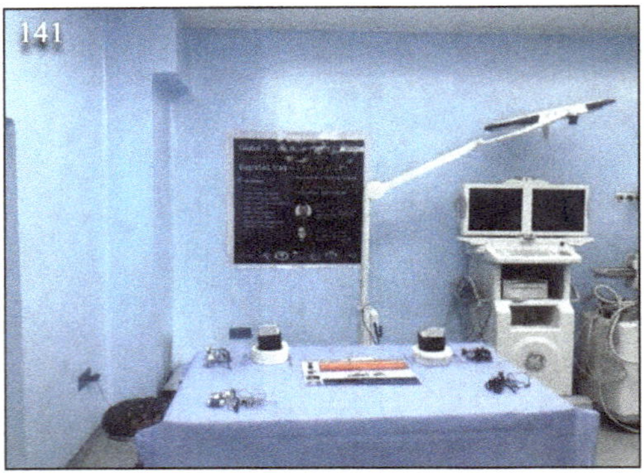

141

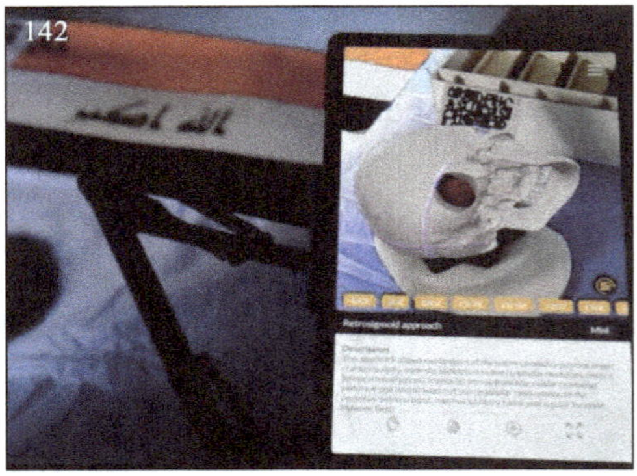

142

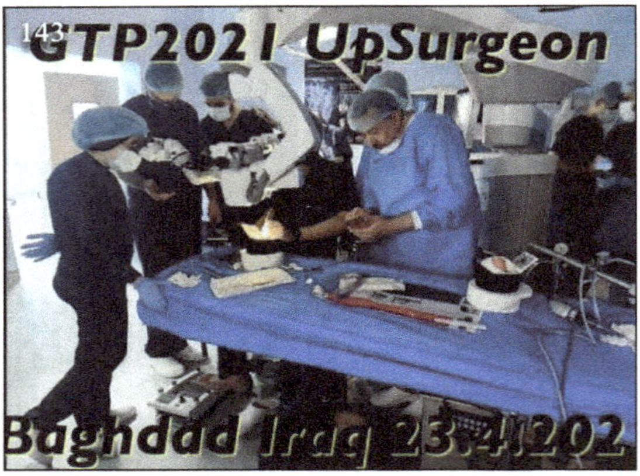

143

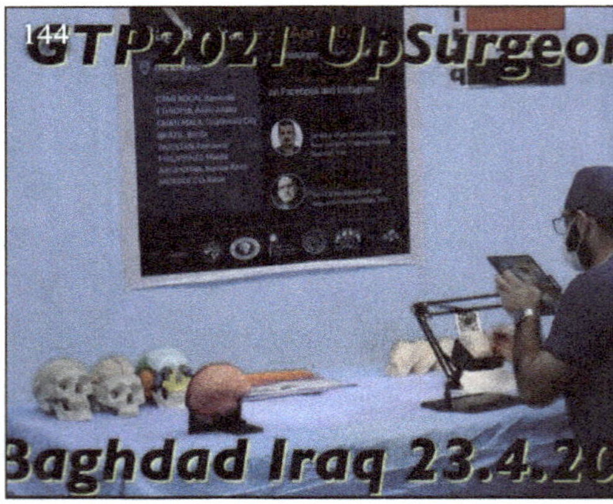

144

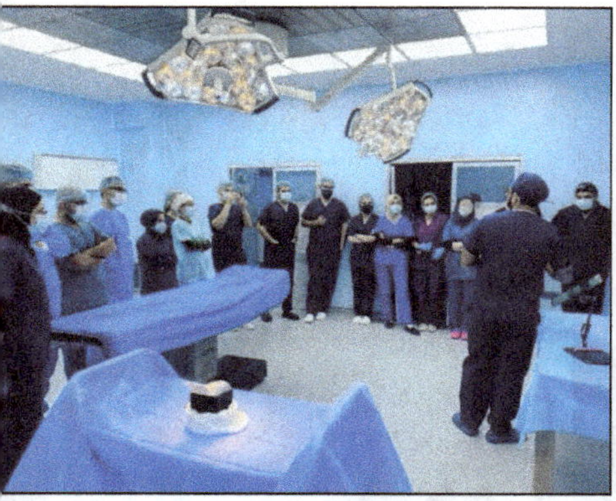

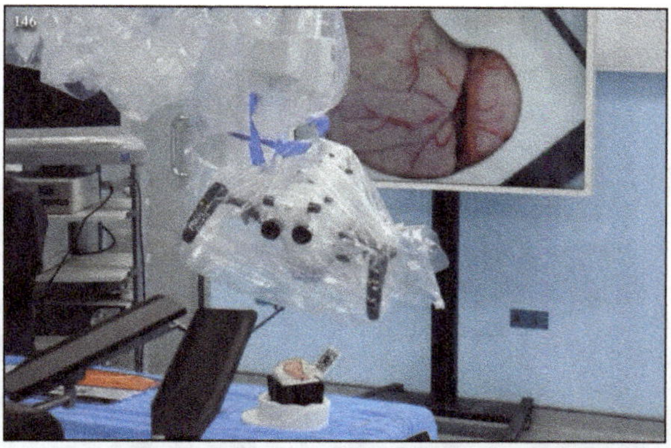
146

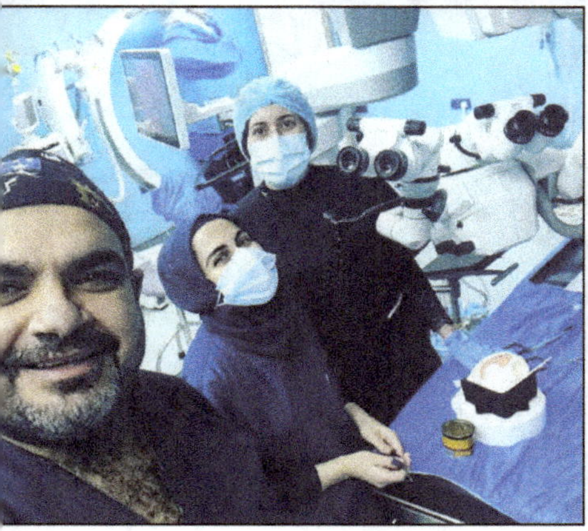

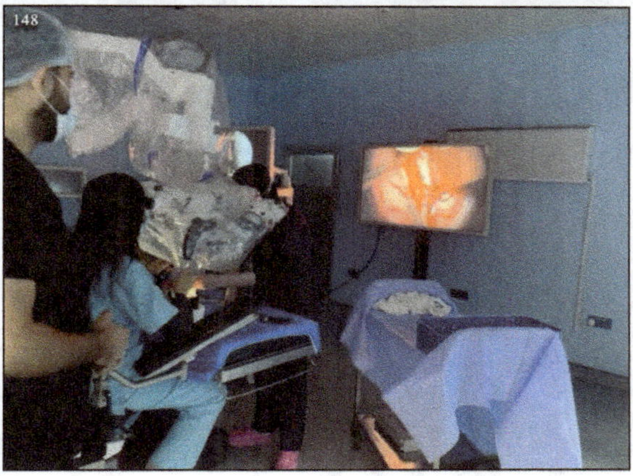
148

Date: Jan 4th 2022

Occasion: Collaboration with Dr. Hossam

Location: Online and Al-Moyad Private Hospital

149

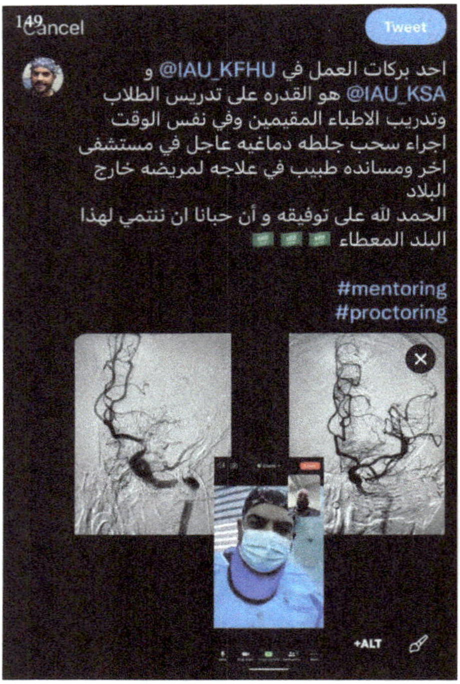

150

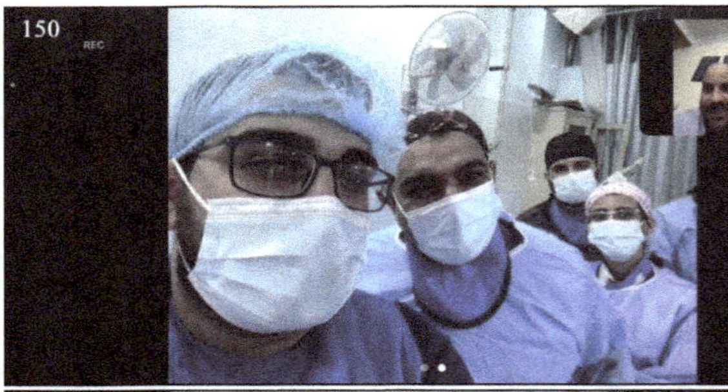

151

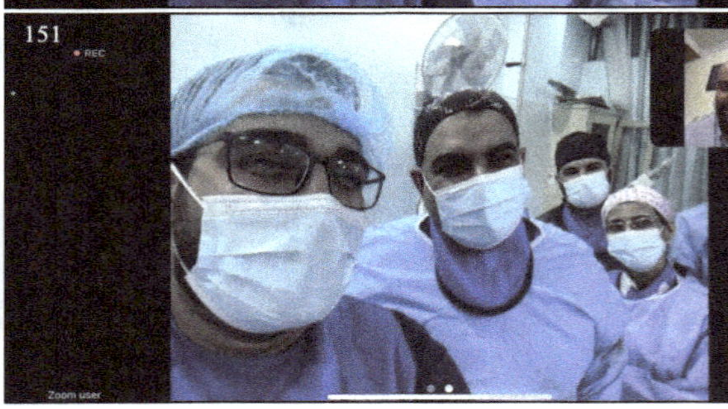

152

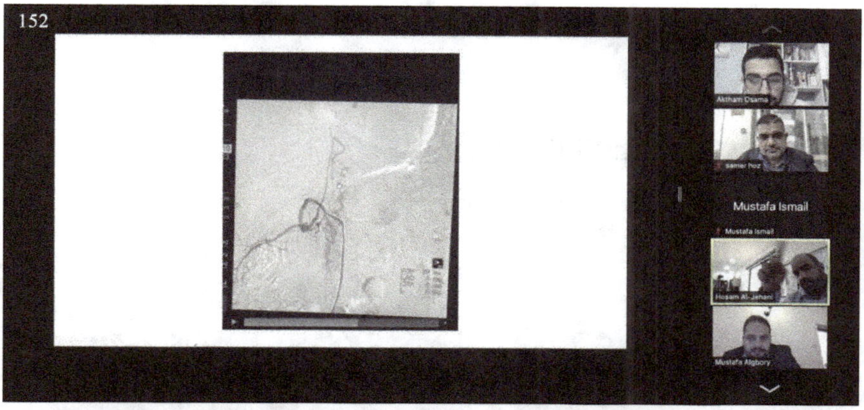
Mustafa Ismail

153

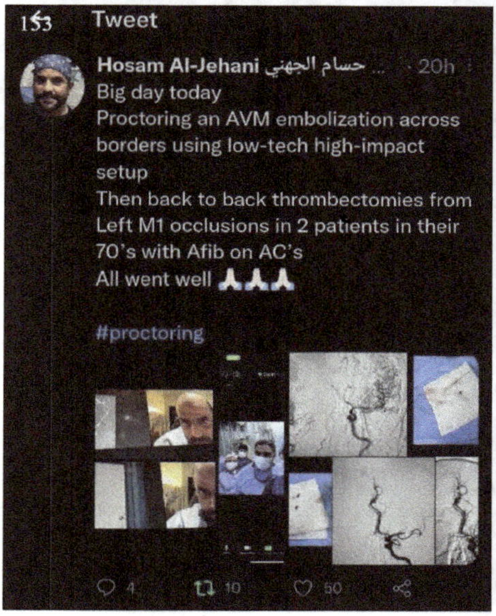
Tweet
Hosam Al-Jehani حسام الجهني ... · 20h
Big day today
Proctoring an AVM embolization across borders using low-tech high-impact setup
Then back to back thrombectomies from Left M1 occlusions in 2 patients in their 70's with Afib on AC's
All went well 🙏🙏🙏
#proctoring
4
10
50

154

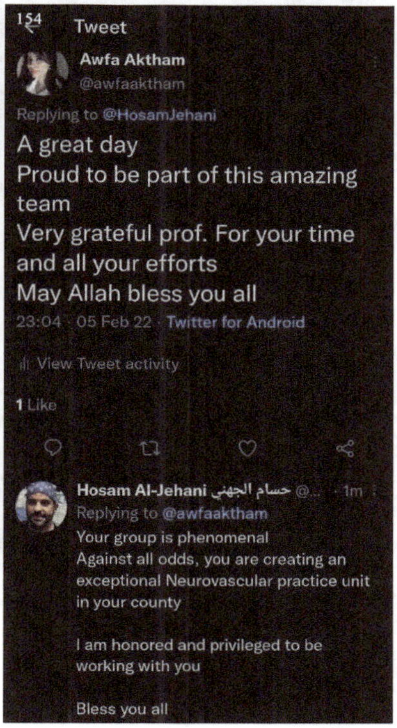
Tweet
Awfa Aktham
@awfaaktham
Replying to @HosamJehani
A great day
Proud to be part of this amazing team
Very grateful prof. For your time and all your efforts
May Allah bless you all
23:04 · 05 Feb 22 · Twitter for Android
View Tweet activity
1 Like
Hosam Al-Jehani حسام الجهني @... · 1m
Replying to @awfaaktham
Your group is phenomenal
Against all odds, you are creating an exceptional Neurovascular practice unit in your county
I am honored and privileged to be working with you
Bless you all

Parts of some mentee's Favorite moments

Mohammed S. Al-Baldawi

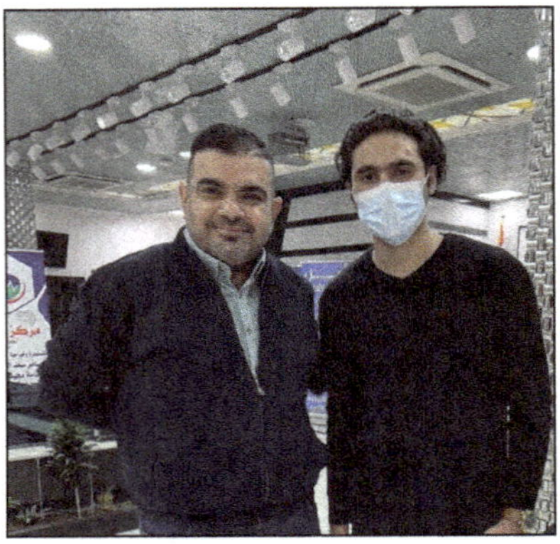

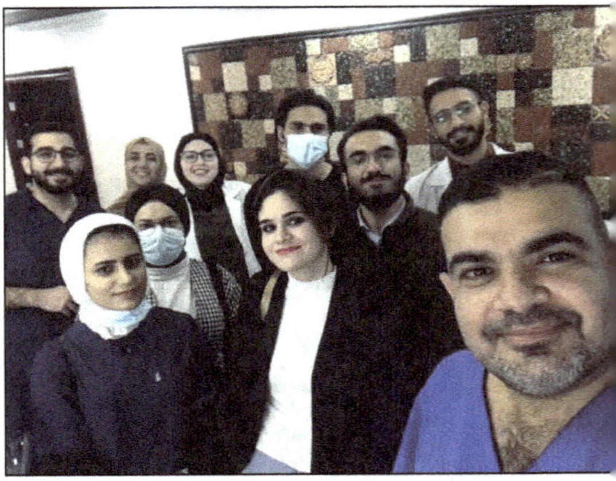

Date & Occasion:

A&**B**: Saturday, 26 February 2022,

First meeting with Dr. Hoz & his final surgery in Baghdad

Caption:

A: The first meeting with Dr. Hoz will always remain the most meaningful to my heart. One of the unforgettable moments was when Dr. Hoz told me:

"I'm proud of your passion, Ibni. I will help you achieve your goals—keep going."

B: It was also his final surgery in Baghdad—a true gift where I learned lessons that stayed with me for life. It was also an honor to meet my fellow mentees, to get to know them, and to share this journey together. Truly a memory to keep. Thanks to everyone who made this blessing possible.

Aanab O. Abdulameer

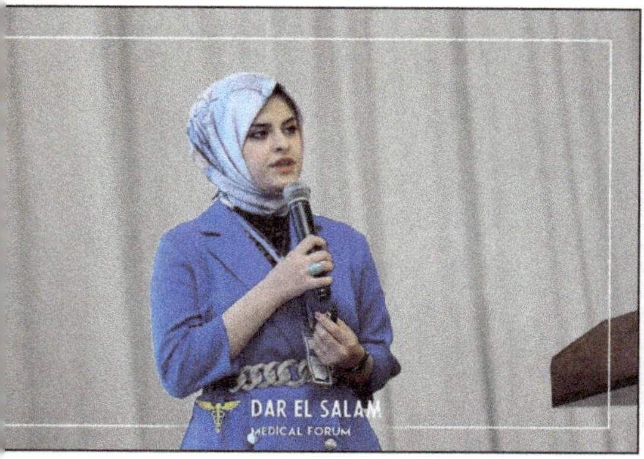

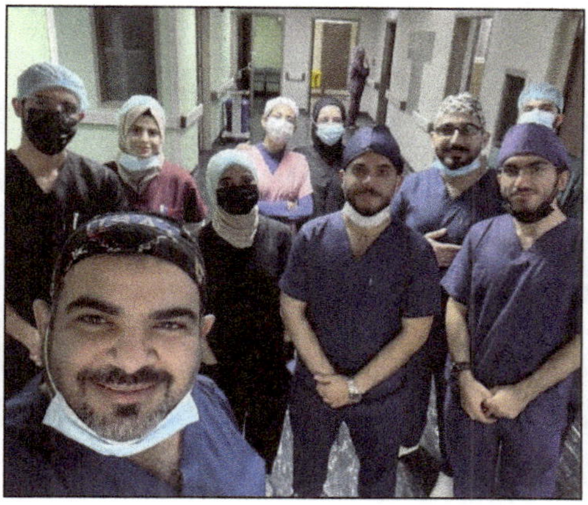

e & Occasion:

n dar al salam medical forum at Iraqi hunting club

August 2023After presenting my 1st case report (impact of dome projection on operative steps during clipping of a ruptured posteriorly directed PCOM aneurysm)

n Ghazi al harriri teaching hospital

of December 2021
n case report impact of dome projection on operative steps during clipping of a ruptured pure posteriorly directed PCOM ırysm.

tion:

During this moment I realize that in neurosurgical field, confidence isn't about having all the answers—it's about asking right questions, staying committed to learning, and standing strong in the face of uncertainty. If you are here, you are able. You are worthy. And the world needs what you have to offer."

s we know that each neurosurgeon should periodically reconsider his or her personal operative environment to had a d performance but in this day I learn a new concept which is (guest neurosurgeon) and how it's important to had ibility and rapid adaptation with new operative environment

is journey of mentorship, we reaffirm that neurosurgery is not confined by walls or titles, but thrives in the collective mitment to healing and learning

Ali M. Neamah

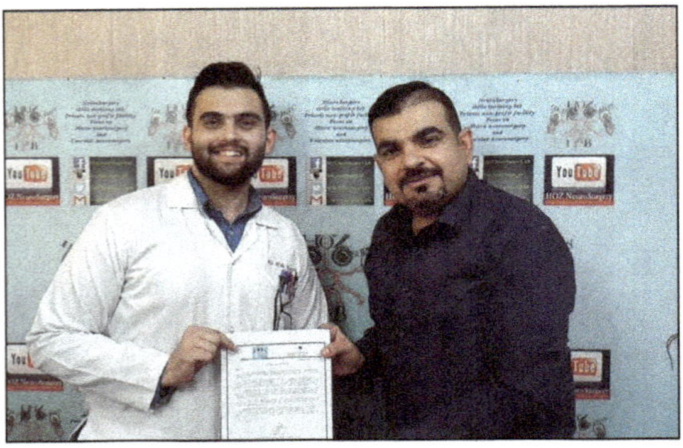

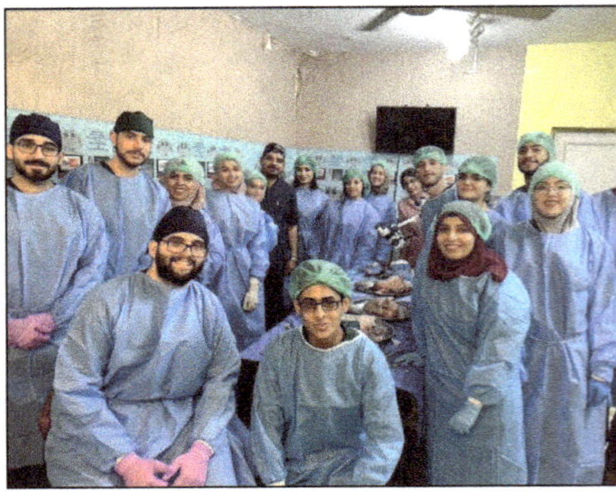

Date & Occasion:

A: A proud moment receiving a certificate of appreciation from my mentor — a symbol of a journey that shaped not just my surgical skills, but my character.

B: With my fellow mentees during the 2019 Neurosurgical Mentorship Program at the Neurosurgical Teaching Hospital

Muhammed S. Al-Shadeedi

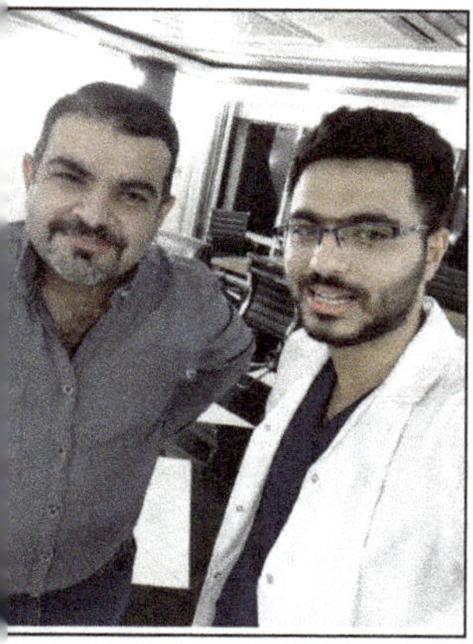

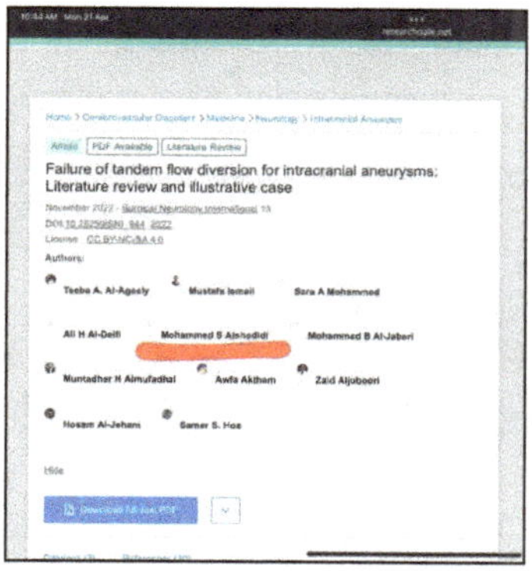

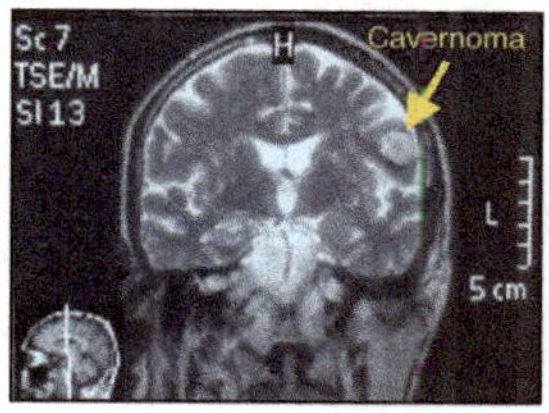

te & Occasion:

st experience in the operating room with 3mmi Samer, Broca's cavernoma

h of July, 2021

To Teach Is To Learn Twice

Joseph Joubert (1754–1824)

www.ingramcontent.com/pod-product-compliance
Lightning Source LLC
LaVergne TN
LVHW022158200926
848481LV00006B/1783

* 9 7 9 8 2 1 8 7 1 5 5 7 1 *